# HEART ATTACK ...
# OR INDiGESTiON
# ARE YOU AT RiSK?

## ROBERTO P. MEDiNA, MD

Published 20 September 2013

ISBN: 149213550X

ISBN-13: 978-1492135500

# CONTENTS

# Foreword

## A Personal Statement

In this book, I will try to answer some of the most frequent questions I hear in my everyday practice: Is my chest pain a sign of an impending heart attack? My doctor told me it is just stress; may stress precipitate a heart attack? Do I need a second opinion? Is my shortness of breath a sign of heart disease, or bad lungs? Is my fatigue just a normal sign of aging? Am I at risk to suffer a stroke? How can I prevent having a heart attack, or a stroke? Am I going to die young, like my father? I hate to take pills; do I really need to take medications for blood pressure, or for cholesterol? How about natural products, diet and exercise? Do I need an invasive procedure? Which one, balloon angioplasty, stent, or something else? What exactly is a balloon angioplasty anyway? Is it true that it was invented in Europe, on somebody's kitchen table? Read on, we are going to touch on these subjects and many more, and try to explain in layman's terms some of the issues related to your cardiovascular health, and how to prevent and treat cardiovascular disease.

What qualifies me to answer these questions? Well, I am a practicing cardiologist, seeing patients referred with just these problems every day. When I see my patients, I make a point to know about their fears and anxieties, not only their symptoms. And we together work out a plan of action in every case, suggest simple solutions when possible, or work on the ways to find out the answers with more sophisticated means when necessary. I am a clinical and invasive-interventional cardiologist, involved in diagnosing, preventing and treating cardiovascular disease for close to 30 years now. I do most of the in-office testing myself, and I do hospital based procedures as well, such as angioplasty and stent implantation. I have the means to get to know your heart in and out, and I know the answers are frequently not as complicated as they appear.

Cardiac disease is the number one killer of both men and women both in the USA and globally. Of the many diseases that affect us, atherosclerosis causes almost one third of all deaths in the industrialized world. This killer doesn't show signs of abating, but it can be prevented and controlled. We will go through the symptoms of heart disease, and the different treatments available, as well as the prevention measures we should be all considering, such as controlling our risk factors. We will review those risk factors, and how to manage them.

What prompted me to write this book is that there is a great deal of confusion "out there" about many of these subjects, and there are powerful interests that want to keep it that way. I think by putting these thoughts in writing, I will be able to reach a broader audience, and hopefully help more people than I would be able to do in my practice. The information contained here is not meant to substitute for a consultation with your doctor, but it may help you to ask the right questions.

This is not a technical book, and I will try to avoid discussing a lot of statistics and technical details. The discussions about the various subjects are based on my informed opinion. I try to keep up to date with the data, but I always try to filter it down through the sieve of my personal experience for the benefit of my patients. I will try to do the same in this book, and present the subject in a highly understandable way. Remember that you alone are ultimately responsible for your health, and you are to make your own decisions. Having said this, it is important that whatever decision you make be an informed one. I hope this book will help guide you to make the right decisions. This is not as easy as it sounds. The information is readily available these days, sometimes even too much information. It is my impression that this information overload, in newspapers, magazines, TV and the internet frequently leads to muddy the waters, and to make the right decisions, we frequently need a guide to help us navigate. It is my hope that this book will be that guide, when it comes to your cardiovascular health.

A personal note: over 40 years ago, my stepfather, who was in his sixties at the time, started having some chest pain. His doctor had prescribed nitroglycerine for him; a little tablet that placed under the tongue gets absorbed very quickly in the circulation and relieves the chest pain. This worked well for months, but one evening, the chest pain would not go away, and became more severe. The doctor came to the house the next morning with his portable electrocardiography machine, and told us that he had suffered a heart attack. He told my stepfather to stop taking the nitroglycerine, stop smoking and keep in bed rest. And to call if he had any more problems. I was a first year medical student at the time, and doubting that this was the best treatment for a heart attack, asked a cardiologist friend for advice. He also came to the house, and confirmed the diagnosis. His advice was that he be admitted to a coronary care unit, where his heart rhythm could be monitored, and where a drug called lidocaine could be administered intravenously to prevent life threatening heart rhythm disturbances that frequently occur during or after a heart attack. That was it. That was the state of the art at the time. Cardiac catheterization had been already invented, but was not in widespread use, and especially not indicated for the acute treatment of heart attacks, as balloon angioplasty had not been invented yet. Although the mechanism of a heart attack, namely the occlusion of a coronary artery by a clot had been already described, there was no way to dissolve the clot or reopen the artery, and it was common belief that nitroglycerin under these circumstances could be harmful by lowering the blood pressure.

Had his heart attack occurred 10 years later or so, he would have been taken to the hospital by a specially equipped ambulance, given nitroglycerine in the vein rather than stopping it, and probably taken to the cardiac catheterization laboratory right away. There, after a diagnostic angiogram, he would have received a powerful medication such as streptokinase in the occluded coronary artery itself. These so-called a thrombolytic agents where very effective, and a few years later it was discovered that they were just as effective if injected in a vein, obviating the need for immediate cardiac catheterization. This treatment with intravenous thrombolytic agents, used with good results for many years is still used in underdeveloped countries where cardiac catheterization is not widely available. The problem with this treatment has been that of severe bleeding complications, and it has been supplanted by acute balloon angioplasty and stent implantation supplemented by various pharmacological agents, as the universally accepted best treatment for a heart attack. The aggressive treatment protocols used today save many lives, and help preserve the heart function in the survivors of heart attacks. We will review all this and much more in the pages of this book, so don't worry if you didn't understand exactly what I just described. I just wanted to exemplify the rapidly evolving state of our knowledge in cardiology. Similar advances have been made in the diagnosis and treatment of many conditions presenting with chest pain, and in the following pages we will review the state of the art in the diagnosis of chest pain, how to prevent heart disease, what diagnostic methods we use, and how do we treat the various conditions that present with this symptom.

Incidentally, my stepfather refused to go to the hospital and survived his heart attack without the benefit of the "modern medicine" of the time. Unfortunately, he continued smoking, and died of lung cancer some 10 years later. I would like to dedicate this book to his memory, as he was responsible for stimulating my curiosity about heart disease that guided me along this career path. I hope this little book will help people like him to better understand their symptoms, and what to do about them.


RPM, May 2013

# Chapter 1

## Heart Attack or Indigestion? Assessing the Risk

---

*QUICK GUIDE*

*In answering the question posed in the title of this book, first we have to consider the risk factors for developing coronary artery disease. These risk factors are harbingers of atherosclerosis, and if you have the misfortune of having several of them, your risk of developing a heart attack is much higher. The good news is that most of them are manageable, and by lowering your risk profile, you can be in control. Being a **male** or a **post menopausal female**, as well as being **older**, represent non-modifiable risk factors. Same for a **family history** of early heart attacks or strokes. Beyond these, all the other risk factors described in this chapter are manageable. They range from lifestyle issues, such as **smoking** and being **sedentary**, to severe illnesses such as **diabetes and high blood pressure**. **Obesity** is a risk factor by itself, and is associated with the other risk factors, such as diabetes and hypertension. Ask your doctor how many of these risk factors do you have, how severe they are, and what to do to manage them. Then you have to develop goals that you can actually reach, and a reasonable timetable. In chapter 9, we will come back to these issues in more detail.*

*For more information or to contact the author, visit <http://www.tampacardiologist.com>.*

---

Without any doubt, chest pain *(see Fig 1)* is the number one complaint in a cardiology practice, closely followed by shortness of breath and palpitations. Each of these symptoms may represent a serious health problem, sometimes even life-threatening, but they are just as frequently related to non-cardiac factors. How can we tell if a chest pain is a serious problem or not, could it be the harbinger of a heart attack or just a case of indigestion? First of all, we look at the whole person, and not just the symptoms. Any symptom is more likely to be a serious problem if the person has a high risk profile to start with. What do we mean by "risk profile?" Basically, your risk profile depends on how many of these risk factors you have. Of course, having established atherosclerotic disease in an area already suggests that it may develop in other areas as well. For example, having pain in the calf muscles of the legs when walking is called intermittent claudication. This is associated with peripheral arterial disease (PAD), or atherosclerotic blockages of the arteries in the legs. There is a strong association of heart disease with PAD, and even though this is not a traditional risk factor, it is a strong predictor of heart disease.

We are going to briefly enumerate some of the most important risk factors here, and in a later chapter we will talk some more about how to prevent the development and progression of heart disease by controlling these risk factors when possible. These are the risk factors:

**Age and gender:** These, along with family history are the pre-determined, non modifiable risk factors. Of

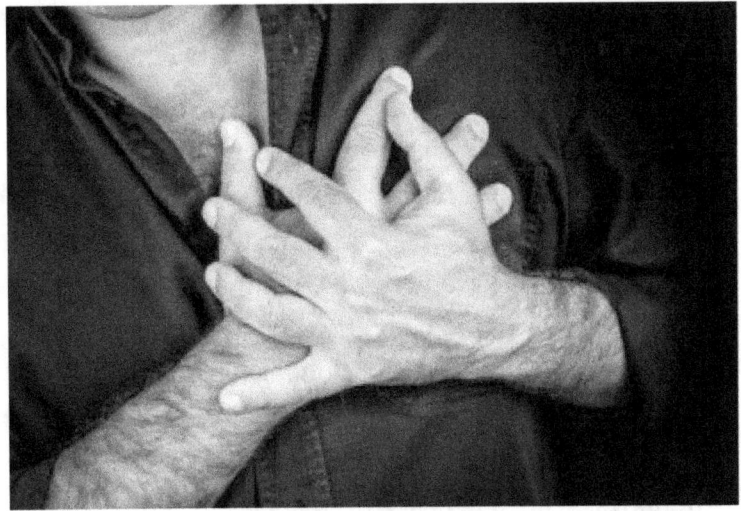

*Fig 1: Chest pain*

course, the age and the gender of the person suffering chest pain matter, as older people have a higher risk of developing heart disease than younger ones, and males have a higher risk of coronary artery disease than females. The gender difference starts to disappear when women become post menopausal, at which time their risk will "catch up" with age matched males. Seemingly, female hormones (estrogens in particular) have somewhat of a protective effect, even though estrogen replacement in post-menopausal women is probably not beneficial. We will review here the traditional risk factors, in chapter 8 we will come back to them and analyze them in more detail.

**Diabetes:** This disease, in the opinion of many experts, is the equivalent of having atherosclerosis of the blood vessels, leading to heart attacks and strokes. If you are diabetic, the risk of heart attack and stoke goes up significantly, and increases even more when is not well controlled. Only strict control may lead to a long life. Of course diabetes is associated with other risk factors, such as obesity, and if you have type II diabetes, strict diet and weight control may "cure" the diabetes. In type II diabetes, which is usually developed in adult life, there is plenty of insulin in the body, but the cells are resistant to its effect, leading to elevated blood sugar, and eventually to vascular complications such as heart attack and stroke, and also peripheral vascular disease of the lower extremities. The diagnosis of diabetes is done with a simple blood test, and the treatment includes diet, weight loss and aerobic exercise, as well as various medications. Oral and more recently injectable medications are used in most cases, and insulin injections are added when necessary. As already mentioned, strict control of diabetes leads to a decrease in the risk of heart attacks and stroke.

**Smoking or any exposure to nicotine:** Smoking is undoubtedly a huge risk factor, not only for coronary artery disease, but also stroke and peripheral artery disease of the lower extremities. I have known very few life-time smokers that did not develop one of these disorders. Fortunately, the incidence of smoking is declining in our country, but not so much in others. Second hand smoke and other forms of nicotine also seem to increase the risk, and are to be avoided. If you still smoke, now is the time to quit. There is plenty of help out there, including support groups, medications, and nicotine replacements, to provide for a "soft landing" for the smoker.

**Hypertension:** This is another major risk factor, especially longstanding hypertension. Don't fret if your blood pressure is elevated one day, it tends to fluctuate throughout the day, and in response to a number of outside stimuli. It is regulated by the autonomic nervous system, so any stress may make it rise, and we have no voluntary control over it. However, if it is elevated most of the time, it needs to be treated. Normal blood pressure is 120/80 or lower, and the lower the blood pressure the longer you can expect to live. Low blood pressure is only a problem if it produces symptoms of lightheadedness or fainting. Hypertension, as diabetes, also goes hand-in-hand with obesity. Salt in the diet also raises blood pressure. Non-pharmacological, natural ways of treating hypertension, include weight loss, aerobic exercise, and salt restriction, and may be sufficient to bring it under control. However, frequently it is necessary to take medications to lower blood pressure.

**Cholesterol and serum lipids:** This issue could fill a whole book, and it is very frequently the main question asked in a cardiology visit. What is the relationship of cholesterol and the hardening of the arteries or atherosclerosis that may eventually lead to a heart attack? We will come back to this subject later in this book, as we discuss the formation of plaques in the arteries (atherogenesis) and the ways to prevent it. There are many ways to fractionate cholesterol in the blood, as there are many molecules that constitute what is measured as total cholesterol on a routine blood test. High cholesterol, and particularly the LDL-cholesterol fraction, is very strongly associated with the risk of developing heart disease and atherosclerosis, as well as stoke. Early research has shown that each percent reduction in cholesterol level, results in a 2 percent reduction in the incidence of coronary artery disease. High triglycerides, another serum lipid, may be associated with increased risk as well. A low saturated or animal fat diet may contribute to lower LDL cholesterol, and a plant based diet may be very effective, even producing regression of atherosclerotic plaque in some cases. Fish oil, specifically omega 3 fatty acids may contribute to improve the lipid profile, and so is exercise and weight loss.

**Obesity:** We mentioned obesity as a contributing factor to other major risk factors, such as diabetes, hypertension and lipid disorder. In addition, obesity by itself is an independent risk factor for atherosclerotic diseases, heart attacks or stoke. Obesity is defined as a body mass index (BMI) of 30 or greater and morbid obesity as a BMI of 40 or greater. The BMI is a relationship between the weight and the height of a person by a simple formula, and there are calculators available on the internet. It is not a totally accurate indicator of body fat, as a muscular person may have a high BMI without being obese, but, if you are not a body-builder, BMI is a good way to estimate body fat. Also, obesity as a risk factor has been questioned recently, after a study has shown that a person with a high BMI may do better when he or she gets sick than a person with a low BMI. This was called the "obesity paradox," and it is explained invoking the common concept that the obese person has more energy reserves, needed to fight illness. This however doesn't mean that obesity is no longer viewed as a risk factor, especially in these times when it is considered an epidemic.

**Family history:** This is one of the strongest predictors of cardiovascular disease, and, unfortunately, it is the one where there is no remedy, we don't get to pick our ancestors, we cannot change our genes. To represent a risk factor, family history has to occur in direct family members, (parents or siblings), and it can be atherosclerotic heart disease, heart attack or stroke, occurring at age 65 or younger for female relatives, and 55 or younger for males. Of course, sometimes heart disease that started at younger age, is not diagnosed until after age 65, in which case it may still be a significant risk factor. Heart disease in second degree relatives or in older parents and siblings is not a recognized risk factor.

# Chapter 2

## What Is Coronary Artery Disease?

*QUICK GUIDE*

*In this chapter, we review the anatomy and physiology of the heart, and how it receives its blood supply through the **coronary arteries**, and how these small but important arteries are at the center of most cases of chest pain. In **coronary artery disease (CAD)**, the coronary arteries become hard and cannot dilate when more blood is needed, and/or develop plaques that limit the blood supply to the heart. We introduce the concept of **atherosclerosis**, and the role of **cholesterol** in the formation of atherosclerotic plaque. We explain how the **"bad cholesterol" (LDL)** promotes the formation of plaque, and the **"good cholesterol" (HDL)** helps in its removal. Ask your doctor what is the likelihood that you already have those plaques, and what testing would he recommend to determine if you have them or not. Also, ask about your cholesterol levels, and if you have "bad cholesterol" (LDL), or "good cholesterol" (HDL). Your doctor may recommend blood tests to determine this, and other details related to your metabolism and the formation of atherosclerosis.*

***For more information or to contact the author, visit http://www.tampacardiologist.com.***

**Coronary artery disease (CAD):** To understand CAD, we have to review briefly the anatomy and physiology of the heart and the coronary circulation. The heart is basically a pump powered by muscle that contracts and relaxes with each cardiac cycle, normally between 60 and 100 times a minute. It has two upper chambers, the right and left atria; two lower chambers, the right and left ventricles; and four valves *(see Fig 2)*. The right and left heart chambers are in reality two separate pumps, the right ventricle giving rise to the pulmonary circulation and the left ventricle to the systemic circulation *(see Fig 3)*. The left ventricle is a thick-walled, powerful pump, pushing the blood into the aorta, that then distributes it throughout the system (hence the name of systemic circulation). The blood, depleted of oxygen by the various tissues and organs of the body, returns to the right atrium that then empties into the right ventricle. The right ventricle, much thinner and weaker than the left, only has to pump the blood to the lungs where it receives oxygen (the pulmonary circulation). The oxygenated blood then returns to the left atrium and from there to the left ventricle, completing the circuit. The blood vessels carrying blood from the heart to the tissues (or the lung) are called arteries. Those that return the blood to the heart are the veins. The main pumping chamber therefore is the left ventricle, requiring a lot of oxygen to do its work.

The heart, in spite of being full of blood, does not receive its oxygen from this blood, but through some small but very important arteries on its surface: these are

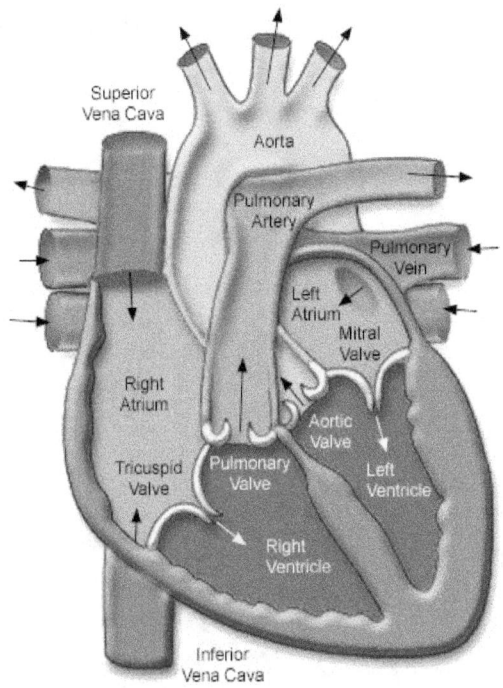

*Fig 2: The heart*

the coronary arteries *(see Fig 4)*. They have their origin in the aorta, the main blood vessel leaving the left ventricle, and distribute throughout the heart muscle, most abundantly in the left ventricle, as it requires more oxygen. There are two major coronary arteries rising from the aorta just after leaving the heart. They are the right coronary artery and left coronary artery. This latter one is usually the biggest and most important one. The left main coronary artery, referred to as the "widow maker," (its occlusion is often fatal), gives off two mayor branches, the left anterior descending (LAD) and the left circumflex (LCF). Each one of these three principal arteries (LAD,

LCF and right coronary artery or RCA) gives rise to several branches on the surface of the heart, and eventually into the heart muscle itself.

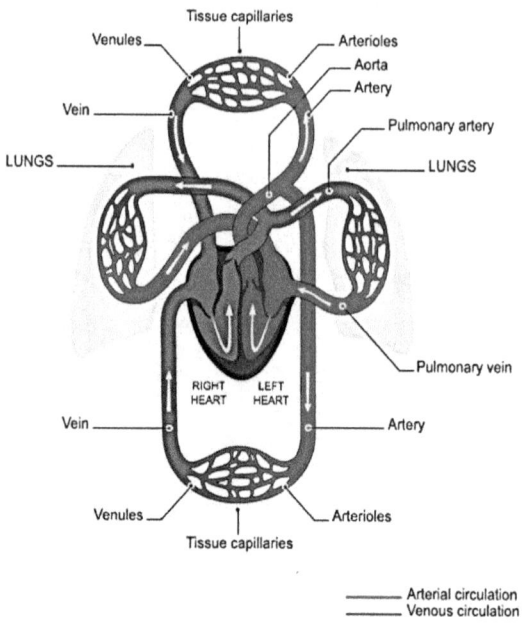

*Fig 3: The circulation*

Normally, these coronary arteries are able to deliver oxygenated blood to the heart muscle, increasing the volume as needed. So, when we get ready to exercise or fight, or in response to stress, the autonomic nervous system sends a signal to the coronary arteries to dilate, to be able to deliver oxygen to the heart that needs to work extra hard. Interestingly, the same branch of the autonomic nervous system that dilates the arteries, makes the heart beat faster and stronger, makes the pupils of the eyes dilate, makes the digestion slow down or stop to divert blood to the muscles and the heart itself, etc, a phenomenon that occurs in many animals in response to perceived danger, called the "fight or flight" response. All this occurs without our conscious intervention, hence the name of autonomic nervous system. It is the same response that makes the hair in the back of the cat stand up, and the coronary arteries in our hearts (and that of most vertebrates) dilate increasing the blood flow to the heart muscle. Of course, when these arteries are hardened by atherosclerosis, this vasodilator response is impaired.

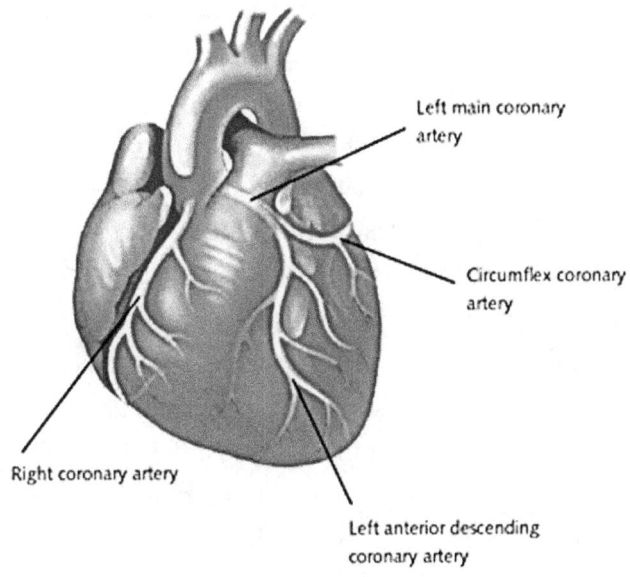

*Fig 4: Coronary arteries*

**Atherosclerosis and cholesterol:** So, what happens in CAD at the microscopic level in the coronary arteries, what is atherosclerosis and how does it develop? What is the link between atherosclerosis and cholesterol? The normal artery is covered inside by a "skin," a thin layer of cells called endothelium, covering the inner-most layer called the intima *(see Fig 5)*. The middle layer, called the media, is mostly composed of muscle cells, able to constrict or dilate the artery, as we discussed before. The outside layer is called the adventitia. When atherosclerotic plaques start to form, lipids start to deposit under the endothelium and in the media, in the form of cholesterol-laden cells; this earliest visible sign of atherosclerosis is called a **fatty streak**. This occurs early in life: by the age of 20 many of us already have some fatty streaks, as demonstrated many years ago in autopsies of young soldiers that died in the Korean war. Next, these cells will concentrate in certain areas, forming raised lesions in the arterial wall; this is what is called the **atherosclerotic plaque**. These plaques contain fibrous tissue and a cholesterol core. As cholesterol when concentrated in this manner is poisonous to the surrounding cell material, these cholesterol-laden cells tend to die from the core out, eventually leading to the rupture of the plaque through the torn endothelium. When this happens, the cholesterol-rich core in contact with the circulating blood activates the circulating platelets, and eventually leads to the formation of a clot, that in turn may lead to a heart attack, or myocardial infarction. How does the cholesterol get into the arterial wall? Packed in particles of LDL, or low density lipoprotein, that help the cholesterol cross the endothelium. Hence the name of "bad cholesterol" given to LDL-cholesterol. How can cholesterol be excreted out of the arterial wall? Packed in particles of HDL, or high density lipoprotein, hence the name of "good cholesterol" given to HDL-cholesterol. These particles then take the cholesterol back to the liver for its disposal. So, atherosclerosis results from a balance between LDL that promotes the deposition of cholesterol, and HDL that promotes its removal. Measures that can change this balance favorably, such as diet, exercise and medications, may lead not only to the decrease in the formation of plaque, but also its removal once formed.

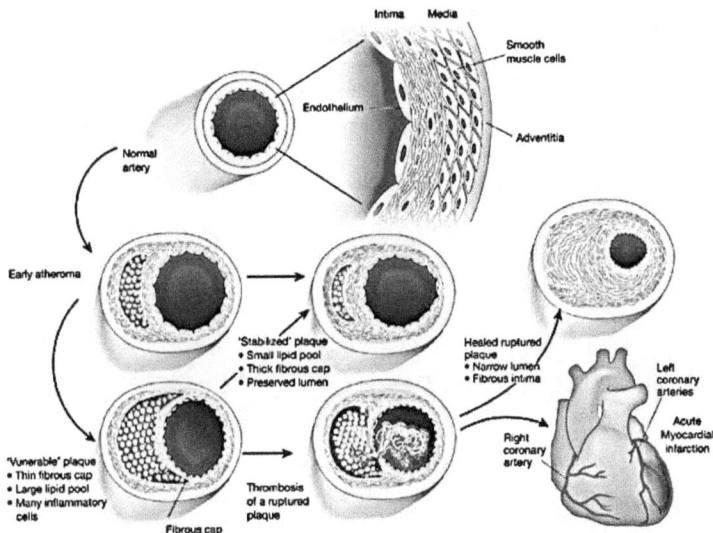

*Fig 5: Plaque formation and rupture*

When the cholesterol-rich core in the atherosclerotic lesion leads to the death of the surrounding cells, this not always results in the rupture of the plaque. Sometimes, it leads to a form of healing, with proliferation of the muscle cells, deposit of fibrous tissue, and the formation of raised plaques. These plaques, when they obstruct the artery by around 70% or more, lead to a significant decrease in normal blood supply. In addition, the diseased coronary arteries containing these atherosclerotic plaques harden and lose their flexibility. These hardened arteries cannot respond normally to the vasodilator stimuli of the autonomic nervous system, and therefore, are unable to supply the needed increase in blood and oxygen to the heart muscle when we exercise, for example. This lack of oxygen in the heart, occurring with effort, exercise, or sometimes stress, is called **angina pectoris** or simply **angina.**

# Chapter 3

## Chest Pain: Is It the Heart or Something Else?

*QUICK GUIDE*

*This chapter looks at the various causes of chest pain, those that may lead to a heart attack, and those that are due to something else. We define words that we use for cardiac chest pain, such as **myocardial infarction, angina pectoris and acute coronary syndrome**. We talk about the quality and location of the chest pain that may point to a cardiac origin, and the changes on the electrocardiogram in these situations. Then, we consider the non-cardiac causes of chest pain, such as **GERD** (gastro-esophageal reflux disease) and gallbladder diseases such as **cholecystitis**, lung problems such as **pulmonary embolism**, and other cardiac and non-cardiac causes of chest pain. Chest pain is likely to be a serious problem even if it is not due to CAD, and it always deserves a consultation with your doctor. We will review the methods your doctor will use to evaluate your chest pain in the following chapters.*

***For more information or to contact the author, visit http://www.tampacardiologist.com.***

**Angina, acute coronary syndrome and heart attack:** We experience chest pain as a result of a decrease in the oxygen delivery to the heart muscle, a phenomenon called **ischemia**. There are no pain nerve endings in the heart otherwise; you can stab a person in the heart and it will not hurt (of course it will hurt when the knife goes through the skin and muscles). We will discuss this symptom further, enough to say that chest pain occurring with exercise or effort, when the oxygen demand of the heart is greatest is typical of angina pectoris and a symptom pointing to the diagnosis of significant CAD. When this symptom occurs only with exercise or effort (or sometimes stress), and is promptly relieved with rest or mild medications, it is called **stable angina.** A completely different presentation may occur in some cases. This is the sudden onset of chest pain, occurring either at rest or with exercise, and not relieved by anything. This may happen in a person that had angina with exercise before, or it may be the first manifestation of atherosclerotic heart disease. Here the mechanism is different, and it frequently involves the rupture of an atherosclerotic plaque in a coronary artery, as we saw above. This in turn promotes the deposition of platelets from the circulating blood, which then activates the coagulation of the circulating blood and the formation of a blood clot in the artery. If the resultant blockage of the artery is partial, the person is said to have **unstable angina** or an **acute coronary syndrome.** If on the other hand the blockage of the artery is complete, a **myocardial infarction** or heart attack ensues. So if you have severe chest pain "out of the blue," it may be a heart attack, and has to be treated as such until proven otherwise. That means calling 911 and being transported to the hospital as soon as possible. There is a saying in cardiology: time is muscle. The more time goes by between the occlusion of an artery, and its reopening by mechanical means (angioplasty), the more heart muscle dies, which, to our current knowledge, is irreversible. Acute intervention with balloon angioplasty and/or stent deployment in the affected coronary artery, is the universally recognized best treatment option for a so called **STEMI** (ST segment elevation myocardial infarction, referring to a typical appearance of the electrocardiogram in a person suffering a heart attack, *see Fig 6*), the sooner the better. **Unstable angina**, and the variety of myocardial infarction without ST segment elevation on the ECG (**NSTEMI**, or **NON-STEMI**) are called **acute coronary syndromes (ACS),** and here too, acute intervention is the best choice of treatment, although it is not as emergent as in STEMI, where any delay leads to further death of heart muscle cells and ultimately to loss of heart function. By the way, the same is true for a stroke in terms of loss of brain tissue, but the treatment options are somewhat more controversial, and outside the scope of this book.

So, we have discussed chest pain occurring with exercise or effort, and called it angina pectoris, and we also considered chest pain at rest that, when severe and persistent may represent an acute coronary syndrome or a heart attack. In our discussion we have said nothing yet

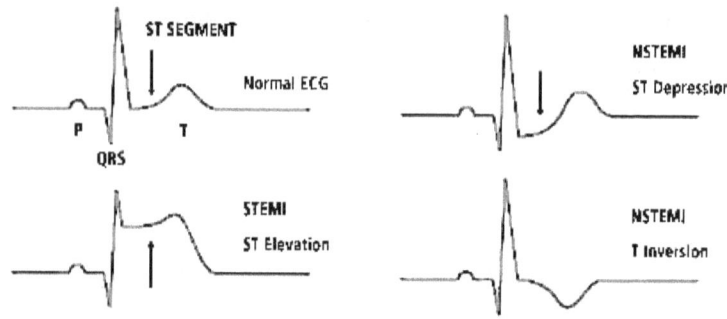

*Fig. 6: ECG in acute myocardial infarction*

about the quality and location of the pain, and this is important. Cardiac chest pain may be located anywhere, but is typically located in the middle of the chest, sometimes a bit to the left of the middle *(see Fig 1)*. It may typically radiate to the left shoulder, or left arm, although it may go to the throat or the jaw, to the back between the shoulder blades, or to the right side instead of the left. I had patients that had teeth pulled thinking they had toothache, when in reality it was angina. The location of the pain does not indicate which side of the heart, or even which coronary artery is involved. It is said that women tend to have more "atypical" symptoms. Sometimes pain in the jaw or arm occurs without chest pain at all; I had a patient that had only pain in the middle finger of the left hand. Any pain above the waist that occurs with exercise or effort and is relieved with rest should be suspicious.

What is the quality of the ischemic pain? As we saw, this results from a decrease in oxygen in the heart muscle.

It is usually an aching type of pain, dull rather than sharp, more like a toothache and less like a stabbing knife. It is typically more severe in cases of heart attack than in simple angina pectoris, and of course, longer lasting. Frequently patients tend to minimize the symptom, as it is not severe. They may think it is a shoulder cramp, or gas pain as it sometimes it gets better with belching. The typical image of the person grabbing his or her chest in pain when having a heart attack is the exception rather than the rule. Frequently patients characterize it as a sensation of tightness. Women try to loosen their bra, thinking it is too tight. Some patients describe a sensation of heaviness, and feel a weight on the chest, "like a ton of bricks."

**Ischemia vs. other causes of chest pain:** Of course, not all chest pain is due to ischemia and it may be unrelated to the heart altogether. I would venture to say that most chest pains are non-cardiac, as there are many tissues and organs in the chest, all with their unique pathology. Sometimes chest pains of a different origin may be mistaken for angina, and treated with nitroglycerin tablets under the tongue. If the pain gets relieved with nitroglycerin, it suggests angina, but of course, it may be coincidental. Also, sometimes painful spasm of the esophagus may be relieved with nitroglycerine as well. I am not going to enumerate here the many possible causes of chest pain, but just mention a few that are frequently mistaken for angina.

**Gastro-esophageal reflux disease (GERD)** is frequent and perhaps the most frequent cause of chest pain. The mechanism is a decrease in the tone of the valve at the entrance to the stomach. After eating the food mixes with the acid secreted by the stomach, starting the process of digestion. In GERD the stomach content is allowed to return to the esophagus as a result of incompetence of the above mentioned valve. This acidic sludge is highly irritating to the lining of the esophagus, causing a chest pain similar to that of angina pectoris. It tends to occur about an hour or two after meals, more frequently when lying down (as gravity will no longer help to keep the stomach contents down). Although angina typically occurs with exercise, GERD may sometimes be provoked by exercise as well, as exercise relaxes the valve between the esophagus and the stomach. To complicate things even more, sometimes nitroglycerine will help relax the esophagus, relieving the pain caused by esophageal spasm, a related disorder. The positional nature of the pain (lying down) and its occurrence after meals and usually at rest, distinguish this pain from angina. It is treated with antacids and medications that inhibit acid production in the stomach, and with the so-called anti-reflux maneuvers, such as elevating the head of the bed and never lying down soon after a meal.

**Costochondritis:** This is another frequent problem causing chest pain. It consists of an inflammation of the joint between the sternum (breast bone) and the ribs, believed to be caused by a viral infection of the cartilage.

The normal breathing movements or taking a deep breath will further irritate this cartilage, causing pain. It is usually sharp and well localized, not dull and diffuse like angina, and it may change with body position or get worse with a deep breath. It lasts for days and sometimes weeks, and it tends to be recurrent. It is frequent in young women. Exercise may make it worse, as we breathe deeper when exercising. It is treated with dry heat applied to the area, and anti-inflammatory medications such as ibuprofen may help. Of course, non steroidal anti-inflammatory medications make the pain of GERD worse if this is what is causing the chest pain.

**Pericarditis and pleurisy.** Another type of pain that gets worse with a deep breath is the so called pleuritic pain, which, if occurring in the area of the heart may be due to **pericarditis**, an inflammation of the tissue covering the heart. This sometimes is relieved by leaning forward while sitting in bed. Of course, pleurisy, which is an inflammation of the layer covering the lungs may produce similar pain, hence the name of pleuritic pain. Frequently pericarditis or pleurisy are benign conditions, caused by a virus, and will heal by themselves or with the help of anti-inflammatory medications. However, they may be due to more severe infections, such as tuberculosis, or may be a sign of malignant disease. Even when pericarditis is viral, it may be dangerous if fluid accumulates around the heart, a phenomenon called pericardial effusion. This may impair the normal functioning of the heart, and it may even be life-threatening.

Other less frequent causes of chest pain include some that are non-cardiac, such as lung diseases, particularly **pulmonary embolism** (blood clots in the lung), that nevertheless require urgent medical attention as they may be life-threatening if untreated. This can be easily diagnosed, and CT angiograms (a form of computerized tomography) of the lung are now customarily obtained in the emergency room for patients presenting with chest pain. Other diseases may involve the large vessels in the chest, such as **aortic aneurysm and dissection**, causing severe pain. An aortic dissection can be fatal. A CT scan will confirm or rule out the diagnosis of aortic dissection.

Abdominal processes, such as gallstones or **cholecystitis**, or even **pancreatitis** may present with chest pain. It is beyond the scope of this book to review every possible cause of chest pain, and of course, it is frequently caused by entirely benign conditions, such as a pulled muscle or indigestion. The message though is that you should never ignore this symptom. Aside from the fact that it may be a serious cardiac condition, such as a heart attack or unstable angina, even when it is not that it may still be serious and even life- threatening.

In summary, during the evaluation of chest pain, there is no substitute for clinical judgment, and most people with chest pain will require medical attention. This is particularly true for a 65 year obese man with diabetes and a family history of early atherosclerosis that present with a dull, aching pain in the chest radiating to the jaw, occurring every time he walks a block. At the opposite end of the spectrum is a young female, with sharp and well localized chest pain occurring at rest, exacerbated by certain body positions and worsened by deep breathing. However, the presentation of coronary artery disease is frequently atypical in women, and the absence of obvious risk factors is not a warranty against serious heart disease. Of course, the physical examination and the electrocardiogram may help to establish the diagnosis, and additional tests may be necessary as well. We will review how we evaluate chest pain in the following chapters.

# Chapter 4

## Non-Invasive Evaluation of Chest Pain

*QUICK GUIDE*

*In this chapter we review the non-invasive tests that your doctor may indicate for you if you have chest pain. From the simple **electrocardiogram (ECG)**, to complex testing using nuclear medicine techniques **(radionuclide stress test)** and computed tomography **(CT) of the coronary arteries** are reviewed and explained in this chapter. The ECG is most useful in the diagnosis of a heart attack. This and the chest X-ray are done routinely, even in the primary care doctor's office and the emergency room. More complex techniques, sometimes including **stress testing** on a treadmill, and other times using imaging techniques such as the **echocardiogram** are explained in some detail here. Some of these tests are expensive and quite involved, and are usually ordered and performed by cardiologists. The **CT angiogram of the coronary arteries** is an excellent non invasive test to define your coronary anatomy, not to be confused with the calcium score, more simple but not as valuable. Ask your doctor which of these tests would he or she recommend for your specific situation. Sometimes it is preferable to go directly to the cardiac catheterization, explained in the next chapter.*

***For more information or to contact the author, visit** http://www.tampacardiologist.com.*

As discussed in the preceding chapter, chest pain may be caused by many different processes, and even after careful consideration of the location and the quality of the pain, we frequently have to proceed with further evaluation to disclose its origin. After a careful physical examination, your doctor may recommend some additional testing. Of course, we take into account all the risk factors discussed in the first chapter to try to decide how far to go with the testing. Some of these tests are simple, inexpensive and easy to perform, but some others are quite involved, expensive and sometimes even risky.

**ECG:** The simplest and most frequently performed test in the evaluation of chest pain is, of course, the electrocardiogram. We will not go here in details about its interpretation, but it is important to know that, as useful as this simple test is in diagnosing a heart attack and many other conditions, it is frequently either normal or non-specific in cases of angina, even in cases when the person may have severe, possibly life-threatening coronary artery disease. CAD frequently remains "silent" for many years, both in terms of symptoms and changes on the ECG. Therefore, we may have severe CAD, with or without symptoms, with or without ECG changes. When chest pain occurs, it is frequently intermittent, and the same can be said about ECG changes. So, having a normal or non-diagnostic ECG in the doctor's office is not by any means an indication of the absence of CAD. In fact, most people with CAD will have a normal ECG. A normal ECG is a strong indication that the person is not having a heart attack, and an abnormal ECG is frequently associated with some form of heart disease. So, it is an important tool, but by no means a diagnostic one. Most internists and primary care doctors are trained to interpret ECGs, and will refer patients with chest pain and an abnormal ECG to the cardiologist. However, it cannot be emphasized enough, that, if the clinical suspicion is high, a normal ECG is not enough to rule out significant CAD.

**Chest X-ray:** This is also a simple and inexpensive test and, even though is useless to identify significant CAD; it is invaluable to rule out other causes of chest pain. Some of these, such as the presence of a dangerous dilatation of the main blood vessel in the chest called an aortic aneurysm, may be suggested by a simple chest X-ray. Rupture or dissection of an aortic aneurysm is a life-threatening emergency. Other causes of chest pain, such as a hiatal hernia which is a rather benign slippage of part of the stomach into the chest, may be diagnosed on a chest X-ray. Also, of course, there are a number of lung conditions such as pneumonia that may cause chest pain. A chest X-ray may identify other conditions related to the heart, such as congestive heart failure and cardiac malformations. Congenital malformations of the heart are outside the scope of this book. However, CAD sometimes remains silent until it results in congestive heart failure, and the chest X ray helps to identify this serious condition. So, this is a very useful screening test, which is obtained routinely in the emergency room or at the primary care doctor's office in all cases of chest pain or related symptoms.

**Blood testing:** It is important to know that there is no blood test that would be diagnostic of CAD. Nevertheless, blood testing is frequently performed, and it can be very useful. For example: we discussed that anginal chest pain is caused by a lack of oxygen supply to the heart. Although this is most frequently related to the narrowing of the coronary arteries due to atherosclerotic plaque, it may also be caused by a decrease in the capacity of the blood to carry oxygen from the lungs to the heart. This in turn is most frequently caused by anemia, which would certainly show up on a simple blood test.

Other ways that a blood test may be useful, is to rule out a recent heart attack. As opposed to CAD, a recent heart attack can be diagnosed by a blood test frequently obtained in the emergency room. There are certain so called biomarkers, that if present in the blood indicate damage to heart muscle cells, which is the definition of myocardial infarction (MI) or heart attack. If these biomarkers such as troponin are present in the blood of a person with chest pain, it is an indication for immediate admission to the hospital.

Yet another of the many uses of blood testing is to define the risk profile of a person. Chest pain in somebody with elevated cholesterol or an unfavorable lipid profile is more likely to represent CAD. Even if this turns out to be a false alarm, the lipid profile may identify who is a candidate for early or so called "primary" prevention, to avoid the development of atherosclerotic disease, or halt its progression if already present.

**Exercise stress testing:** This is another simple and inexpensive screening test, frequently but not always performed by cardiologist either in the clinic or in the hospital. It is indicated as a screening tool in people with an increased risk profile, especially if they have chest pain. It is done by walking on a treadmill according to an established protocol. The vital signs and the electrocardiogram are continuously monitored during and after exercise. It starts out slowly, and both the speed and the incline of the treadmill are increased every three minutes, until a certain heart rate is achieved. The desired target heart rate varies by age (the higher the younger the person is) and the predicted exercise time on the treadmill varies by age. Not everybody reaches their targets, and a person who is not in good physical condition may reach the target heart rate sooner than an athletic person. All of this is analyzed to reach a conclusion. It is called a functional test, because it gives us information about the functional status of the person. The ECG may be normal at rest, but, if the coronary arteries are obstructed or lack the capacity to dilate with exercise, it will show certain changes with exercise that may be diagnostic. If these changes are accompanied with chest pain, the diagnostic accuracy is even higher. An exercise stress test is valuable even in the absence of typical symptoms, as it may disclose so called silent ischemia (lack of adequate blood supply) in people with risk factors for CAD.

As simple as this test is, it is not indicated for everybody. If you are having chest pain at rest, without exercise, especially if your ECG is not normal, your doctor will be reluctant to have you exercise on the treadmill. This is both because it may be dangerous to exercise, and because the exercise ECG would not be diagnostic if the resting one is already abnormal. Depending on other variables, you may be a candidate for a different test, or for admission to the hospital. Of course, if for whatever reason, you cannot exercise you are not a candidate for an exercise stress test. In these cases, there are forms of "chemical" or pharmacological stress tests without the need to exercise, that we will discuss below.

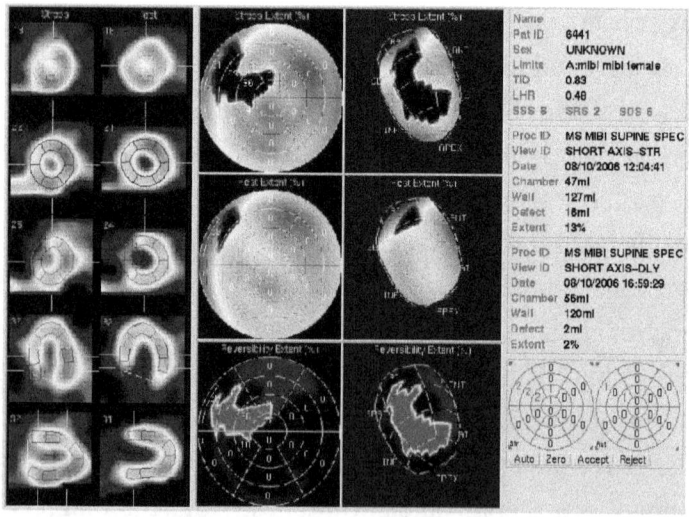

*Fig 7: Radionuclide stress test*

**Radionuclide stress test:** For this test, a radionuclide capable of emitting gamma rays is injected in the vein, and a scan is performed which involves imaging with a gamma-camera over the heart. This is similar to an X-ray procedure, such as a CT scan, but instead of shining the rays through the body, the camera picks up the radiation of the radionuclide injected in the vein. According to how this radionuclide distributes in the heart muscle, the cardiologist can draw conclusions as to the possibility of blockage in one or another coronary artery *(see Fig 7)*. This test is frequently combined with stress testing, in cases when the simple stress test is abnormal or inconclusive. When the person cannot exercise, there is the possibility to perform a radionuclide stress test using a pharmacological agent injected in the vein in lieu of exercise. The imaging part is the same, without the need to walk on the treadmill.

The radionuclide stress test starts with a resting scan, followed by the exercise stress test, and repeat imaging after exercise. By comparing the resting and post exercise scans, conclusions can be drawn about the blood distribution in the heart. Finding an area of decreased radionuclide uptake after exercise that shows normal uptake at rest, means that there is decreased blood supply or ischemia induced by exercise, a strong indication of a narrowed coronary artery. If the uptake at rest and after exercise is equally affected, there may be severe ischemia or a scar of a previous myocardial infarction.

The radionuclide stress test has a much greater diagnostic accuracy than the regular stress test, and is an invaluable tool for the diagnosis of the cause of chest pain. However, it is time consuming and expensive. The radionuclide is produced in a radiopharmacy, and it decays rapidly losing its potency. The dose is ordered for each patient, and it has to be used within a few hours of being produced. The test involves exposure to radiation from the radionuclide, although the half-life is short, just a few hours. The accuracy of the test is not 100% as we are not imaging the coronary arteries, only the uptake of the radionuclide by the heart muscle. In obese patients, or in women with large breasts, there are additional technical difficulties that make the accuracy even lower, because of the interposition of soft tissue. The pharmacological agent used in lieu of exercise has some unpleasant side effects in some patients, although these are usually short-lived. For all these reasons (but of course, mostly for economic reasons), the insurance companies, that frequently require pre-certification if they are to cover the expense, are increasingly denying it, and asking that a different testing modality be used.

**Echocardiography:** This test uses ultrasound to image the heart, which is relatively simple and innocuous. It provides a wealth of anatomical information, but it doesn't have enough spatial resolution to image the coronary arteries. It is used mostly to investigate the dimensions and function of the heart and its various chambers and valves, as it is able to image the heart from different angles in real time *(see Fig 8)*. In addition, it will show if there is fluid around the heart, which may be associated with pericarditis. This inflammation of the tissue around the heart is an important differential diagnosis in the evaluation of chest pain, as we saw above. Aside from this, the value of the resting echocardiogram in evaluating chest pain is limited, and is mostly used to interrogate the heart looking for sign of failure, and to interrogate the four valves *(see Fig 2)* looking for tightening (stenosis), or incompetence (regurgitation). For the evaluation of chest pain, it is performed in combination with the stress test in the stress echocardiogram.

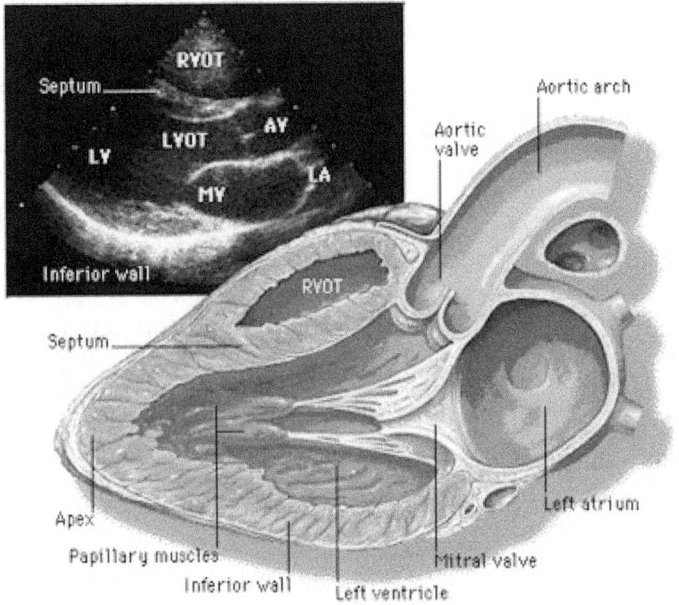

*Fig 8: Echocardiography: parasternal long axis view*

**Stress echocardiogram:** Echocardiography can be used for imaging during the stress test instead of using the radionuclide. This test most frequently includes a treadmill exercise stress test, with echocardiographic imaging before and immediately after the exercise. Then, the resting and stress images are analyzed by the cardiologist side by side. With a proficient technologist imaging a patient who has a favorable body shape and is able to exercise to attain the target heart rate, the diagnostic accuracy of this test is similar to that of a radionuclide exercise stress test. Here, in addition to the traditional echocardiogram, we look at the contraction pattern of the left ventricle before and after exercise to draw conclusions regarding the adequacy of the blood supply. The principle by which it allows us to diagnose coronary artery disease, is that the portion of the heart muscle suffering from poor blood supply, is less able to contract vigorously when stimulated by exercise, and it will show up as a wall motion abnormality on the echocardiogram obtained immediately after exercise.

The stress echocardiogram has several advantages: the resting echocardiogram before exercise provides greater anatomical detail than a radionuclide scan. There is no need to start an intravenous line, as nothing is injected, and, of course, there is no exposure to radiation. Patients that cannot exercise may have their heart rate raised with an IV infusion of the drug dobutamine to simulate exercise, but this is time consuming and negates the main advantages of stress echo: its expediency and simplicity.

**Computed tomography angiography (CTA) of the coronary arteries:** Computed tomography with contrast injected intravenously is able to image the coronary arteries in most people with a high degree of accuracy and, as such, it may replace regular, invasive angiographic procedures. Its main advantage is that it is non-invasive. When compared with other non-invasive modalities, it is the only one that gives a high resolution image of the coronary arteries themselves. For example, it is able to tell us if a coronary artery such as for instance the left anterior descending (LAD) has a 75% narrowing in its mid portion.

CTA is not to be confused with the coronary calcium score, also obtained with CT scanning. This only looks at the presence of calcium in the arteries, being unable to disclose the degree of blockage, or if in fact, there is any blockage at all. Coronary calcium is an indicator of CAD, and as such, the calcium score is a risk factor for the development of blockages, but it will never tell if the chest pain is due to blockages or not, as it does not image the coronary arteries, only the calcium in them. It is a screening test for risk, like the lipid profile that we already considered, or like the level of C-reactive protein in the blood, which is a marker of inflammation. None of these are particularly useful in the evaluation of chest pain.

CTA on the other hand, is very useful as a tool to define the coronary anatomy. The disadvantage is that it does not provide any functional evaluation, and it cannot tell if a certain blockage is responsible for the chest pain. As such, it may be misleading and result in unnecessary angioplasty or stenting procedures. As we will see later, not every blockage needs to be treated with such mechanical procedures, and doing so may be counterproductive. Many invasive-interventional cardiologists, myself included, are prone to suffer from the "oculo-dilator reflex," which assumes that if you see a blockage you need to dilate (perform angioplasty). On the other hand, if a well performed diagnostic radionuclide stress test or stress echocardiogram indicates that there is a problem with the blood distribution to a portion of the heart supplied by a partially blocked artery, and the chest pain did not respond to medical management, this is a much stronger indication to proceed with an angioplasty and stent deployment.

Additionally, CTA is expensive, many times not covered by insurance. It also requires the insertion of an intravenous line, and the injection of a large dose of iodinated contrast material to image the coronary arteries. The exposure to X-rays is substantial as well. Patients with kidney problems that may be made worse by the iodinated contrast material, or those that have already been exposed to X-rays, are not good candidates for this test. Also, the patient needs to have a regular and relatively slow heart rate to be able to scan the coronary arteries, a fast or irregular heart rhythm precludes the use of CTA of the coronaries.

**Holter monitor:** Patients with chest pain frequently complain of palpitations as well, a sensation of irregular heart rhythm, or sometimes too fast or too slow heart rate. This tests monitors the heart rhythm and rate for 24 hours or more, with a take-home portable device. It is very useful to disclose any cardiac rate or rhythm abnormalities, but not so useful in the evaluation of chest pain. However, if the sensation of chest pain is triggered by rhythm abnormalities such an atrial fibrillation, the Holter will be diagnostic in correlating symptoms with arrhythmias. Also, a rapid heart rate can trigger typical angina, by increasing the oxygen demand of the heart muscle.

**Pitfalls of non-invasive testing:** As already mentioned, these so called non-invasive diagnostic tests have some problems in certain patients. The stress test is a simple and inexpensive screening test, but its diagnostic accuracy is low. There are many "false positive" and "false negative" exercise stress tests, where the exercise EKG is plainly misleading. And of course, not everybody can exercise on a treadmill. The imaging tests (radionuclide stress test or stress echocardiogram) improve the diagnostic accuracy of the stress test, but other restrictions may apply, such as in people with a large body size where the imaging is more prone to artifacts. There is also the issue of radiation exposure, or, in the case of CTA, exposure to potentially toxic iodinated contrast material. Each of these tests has a place in the diagnostic arsenal of the physician evaluating a patient with chest pain, but none of them is perfect, and frequently several tests need to be performed to confirm or deny the diagnosis. Sometimes it is more expedient to proceed to the most accurate diagnostic test sooner rather than later.

# Chapter 5

## Invasive Evaluation of Chest Pain

*QUICK GUIDE*

*Here we deal with the techniques that your doctor may use to get a definitive diagnosis of your chest pain.* **Cardiac catheterization** *is performed either after non-invasive evaluation, or directly in some cases. For example, if a heart attack is suspected, only the cardiac catheterization will allow the cardiologist to proceed* **with balloon angioplasty** *and* **stent deployment***, the standard treatment in cases of acute myocardial infarction. If you have chest pain, and the non-invasive tests indicate that it may be due to a blockage in the coronary arteries, your doctor and you will have to decide if cardiac catheterization is indicated. We describe in this chapter the techniques used to gain access to the coronary arteries through the groin, wrist or arm, the possible findings at cardiac catheterization, and the case for and against angioplasty and stenting. You and your doctor should discuss ahead of the procedure the techniques to be used, the risks and benefits, the possible outcomes and the alternatives.*

**For more information or to contact the author, visit** http://www.tampacardiologist.com.

**Cardiac catheterization and coronary angiography:** Despite the many advances in non-invasive testing, as described above, this is still the "gold standard" of testing for the evaluation of chest pain and other cardiac problems. Many insurance carriers these days will ask us to directly proceed with cardiac catheterization after an abnormal stress test (or even without the stress test), as they see many advantages and savings in doing so. I will try to analyze these claims, to allow you to make an informed decision if you are suffering from chest pain.

Let us start with the procedure itself: It consists in the introduction of thin, flexible tubes into peripheral vessels and advance them under X-rays to the heart. In the heart and the coronary arteries we obtain various measurements and angiographic images. The cardiac catheterization laboratory is usually located in a hospital, although it is an outpatient procedure and it can be done in a free-standing facility as well. There is usually no anesthesia involved, and is done under what is called conscious sedation. This doesn't mean, as I have said jokingly, that the patient is sedated and the doctor is conscious, although this is a pre-requisite. Conscious sedation is obtained usually with a combination of sedatives and analgesics injected in the vein, to obtain a significant decrease in the pain and anxiety experienced by the patient, without producing unconsciousness or depression of the respiration. In some cases we use deep sedation, with complete loss of consciousness and amnesia of the procedure. This is not necessary in most cases, as the pain is very mild and the procedure is usually well tolerated. There are no pain receptors in the arteries or the heart, and the only pain experienced by most is during the puncture of the artery and/or the vein to gain access to the circulation. The rest is mostly anxiety, sometimes some palpitations as well. When an angioplasty is performed in combination with the angiogram, there may be some chest pain during the balloon inflation in the coronary artery, as the circulation is transiently occluded and the artery stretched, and this may be managed with additional doses of analgesics. I use morphine sulfate, as it can be titrated to control pain in virtually all cases. Most patients tolerate this procedure quite well.

The arterial system is entered either from the groin (femoral artery), from the wrist (radial artery), or rarely from the arm (brachial artery). In either case, we give some local anesthetic to blunt the pain of the puncture, and then introduce a small sheath the size of a straw, that will serve to advance the catheters. These are thin, flexible tubes, advanced under X-ray (fluoroscopic) control, and they are pre-formed to engage in the structures to image. Most of the time just the artery is entered (left heart catheterization), but sometimes the vein is entered too (right heart catheterization). First he pressures in the various chambers are measured using these catheters and various calculations are made (hemodynamics). Then X-ray images of the coronary arteries *(see Fig 9)* and the heart chambers are obtained, usually imaging the left ventricle (ventriculography). The images of the beating heart and the coronary arteries are recorded in real time on film or hard disk (cine-coronary angiography). The heart structures and arteries have the same density to the X-rays as the surrounding tissues and the blood, so to make them visible we have to inject contrast material in them, via the catheters. Various shapes of catheters are introduced for the different applications, and they can be exchanged through a sheath introduced at the access site. The whole procedure usually takes half hour or less, if no intervention (angioplasty) is performed. Then, the catheters and sheaths are removed, and pressure is applied to make the bleeding stop (hemostasis).

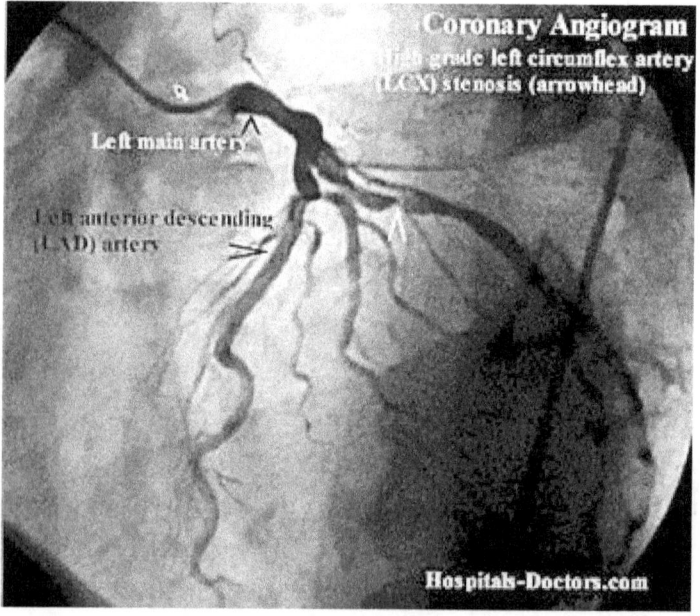

*Fig 9: Coronary angiograph of the left coronary artery*

**Groin (femoral) or wrist (radial) approach?** These are the most frequently used entry sites for all invasive cardiac procedures. Each has advantages and disadvantages, and both have their fans and detractors. In capable and experienced hands, both are equally safe. The radial artery is small, and, along with the ulnar artery provides blood to the hand. The femoral artery in the groin is much larger, and leads from the groin to the leg. Complications with either artery are infrequent. When using the radial artery, we have to make sure that the ulnar artery is patent, assuring continued blood supply to the hand. The reported frequency of radial artery clotting and occlusion during a procedure is variable, as it may not produce any symptoms as long as the ulnar artery is patent. However, this is not a minor complication; it will go undetected until either the patient needs another procedure (and the artery cannot be cannulated) or the ulnar artery fails with dire consequences, which may include the loss of fingers or the whole hand. As these procedures are usually done from the right side, and most people are right-handed, these complications may be profoundly disabling. Fortunately, they are also very rare. The femoral artery is much larger, and thrombosis (clotting) is not a problem. Of course, there are possible complications arising from the groin approach as well, such as the formation of a hematoma (black and blue marks), re-bleeding after hemostasis, and the formation of a so called pseudo-aneurysm due to a weakness in the wall of the artery at the puncture site, resulting from incomplete hemostasis. Usually these complications are self-limited, but sometimes require further intervention. Fortunately, these complications are also rare. The main advantage of the wrist approach is that bed-rest after the procedure is not required, and hemostasis is obtained with a simple device applied to the wrist, not requiring manual or mechanical pressure to stop the bleeding. The groin requires the application of pressure to prevent hemorrhage, and a few hours of bed-rest afterwards. The decision as to which approach to use frequently comes down to the level of comfort of the operator with each modality. When patients hear about the wrist approach they tend to be "sold" on it, without considering the possible complications. I still prefer the groin approach: for me it is quick, it allows me to up-size the catheters if needed, or to use various other tools such as LASER, atherectomy ("shaving" of the plaque), thrombectomy (dissolving a clot with special devices), without having to worry about the size of the catheter needed for the passage of such devices. Of course, sometimes I use a different approach if the femoral artery is unavailable or too deep in extremely obese patients.

How about if the coronary angiogram shows significant CAD, what are the options? First, we have to decide if the symptoms are due to the blockage(s) found. This is an easy decision to make when we are dealing with a heart attack, or a so called acute coronary syndrome (see Chapter 3): here the decision to dilate the vessel is obvious. The dilemma sometimes comes when we are dealing with chronic angina, or a patient with no typical symptoms. This is when a proper functional test provides invaluable information that the cardiac catheterization by itself cannot provide. If the stenosis (narrowing) of the artery is significant, let's say 75% or higher, and there is evidence of ischemia (lack of blood supply) in its territory of distribution, our tendency would be to provide the best available treatment, such as a drug-eluting stent implanted in the involved artery. There may be some controversy in cases of silent ischemia, or if a trial of effective medical therapy has not yet been tried. For these patients, there have been some recent studies that suggest that medical treatment may be preferable to angioplasty. However, I would say that there are very few cardiologists that, if a significant stenosis is found supplying an area of demonstrated ischemia, would tie their hands and let the patient go home without a stent. And I would bet that most patients would not go home happy with medical treatment, knowing that they have a severe stenosis. There are circumstances where the case for angioplasty is even stronger, such as when the LAD (left anterior descending coronary) is involved, or when a severe stenosis is found in any major artery. On the other hand, if a minor branch is involved, or there is no proof of ischemia in the territory of distribution of the involved artery, and in cases where medications have not been tried, we may opt for the non-interventional approach and try medications first.

**Other diagnostic modalities during catheterization:** There are basically two in common use and others on the horizon. The most useful perhaps is the pressure wire that allows the measurement of the pressure distal to the stenosis, along with other parameters. These wires are very thin, similar to the regular guide-wires used to cross the stenosis, and, if intervention is needed, can be used to guide the balloon or stent across the lesion. Once the stenosis is crossed with the wire a medication is injected in the vein or the artery itself to dilate the vessels, which allows the measurement of the **fractional flow reserve (FFR)**, by comparing pressures before and after the injection, proximal and distal to the stenosis. This is a functional measurement, and various trials have shown a correlation of poor outcome when the FFR is decreased below certain level. In this case, stenting is justified.

The other method in common use is **the intravascular ultrasound (IVUS)**. This is an anatomical imaging modality that looks at the artery "from the inside" *(see Fig 10)*. It also uses a thin wire, which in this case has a miniature ultrasound transducer at the tip. It allows a more accurate measurement of the size of the artery and the size of the plaque than the angiogram can provide. We find that frequently that both the artery is larger in diameter than suspected, and that the plaque burden is also larger.

Portions of the artery that appeared relatively normal on the angiogram are sometimes diffusely affected by plaque. The IVUS allows us to look at the arterial wall, not just the lumen (as the angiogram does). Decisions about stenting or not should still be supported on solid clinical grounds, although the IVUS can add valuable information about the diameter and length of the stent to be used, and, if repeated after stenting, it will tell if the stent needs to be dilated more to conform to the artery. Good apposition of the stent to the artery is important for the continued patency of the artery after stenting.

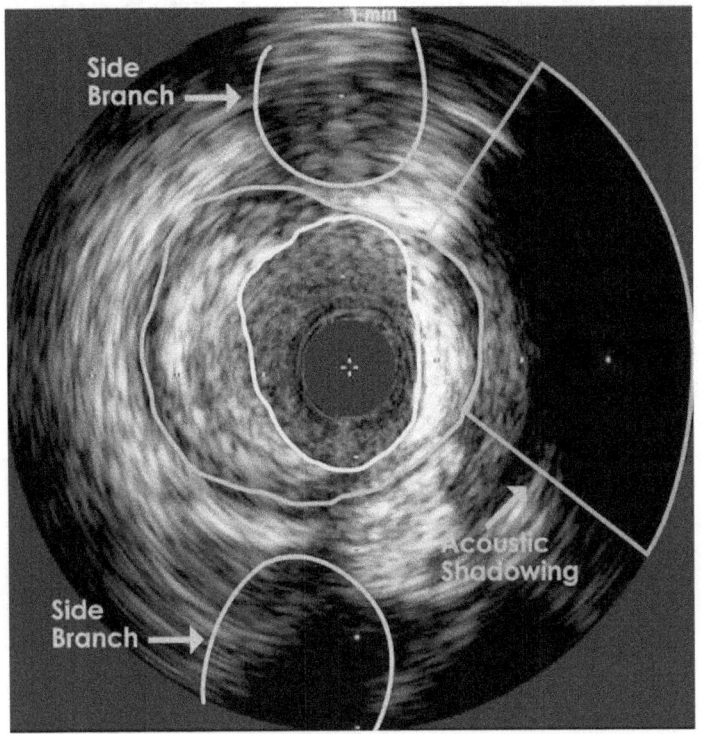

*Fig 10: IVUS showing an eccentric plaque*

There are other imaging modalities: some use color coding of tissue density during IVUS to try to identify which plaque is likely to rupture (vulnerable plaque) leading to an acute event such as a heart attack. The hope is that by targeting these vulnerable plaques for intervention (stent implantation) the outcome can be improved. Then, there are entirely different imaging modalities such as OCT (optical coherence tomography) capable of a much higher resolution image than that obtained with IVUS. As opposed to FFR and IVUS, the exact place of these newer modalities in our armamentarium is still to be defined.

# Chapter 6

## Invasive Treatment of Coronary Artery Disease

*QUICK GUIDE*

*In this chapter we talk about the treatment of CAD with **balloon angioplasty or PTCA**, **stent implantation** and various other invasive treatment modalities such as **atherectomy** and **LASER**. The invention of balloon angioplasty by the charismatic German cardiologist Andreas Gruentzig in his kitchen, and its popularization throughout the world represented a true revolution in cardiology, changing the treatment of CAD forever. The subsequent developments, including the introduction of metallic scaffolds called stents used to keep the artery open after PTCA, are described. We review the advantages of the so-called **drug eluting stents**, where the stent delivers a drug to the artery with the purpose of keeping it open longer. In the following chapter we talk about an unusual but severe complication of stenting, namely the early clotting of the stented area, called **stent thrombosis**. It is very important that you discuss with your cardiologist which procedures is he planning to do during your cardiac catheterization, if he is planning a stent deployment which stent is he planning to use, and what medications you will have to take afterwards and for how long.*

***For more information or to contact the author, visit*** *http://www.tampacardiologist.com.*

So far, we have talked about chest pain and its evaluation, how to individualize such evaluation in light of the various risk factors, and when to proceed to the "gold standard" of diagnostic modalities, the cardiac catheterization. We talked a bit about coronary artery disease (CAD) or the build-up of plaque in the arterial wall, resulting in a lack of normal blood supply to the heart muscle and producing the chest pain symptom that we called angina pectoris. We did not talk much about the medical treatment of CAD, only to mention that it is frequently a viable option, but we will come back to it. Since we just talked about cardiac catheterization and coronary angiography, let us start with the invasive-interventional treatment modalities. Once the diagnosis is obtained and we are convinced that an interventional procedure is needed, we still need to decide which procedure to use.

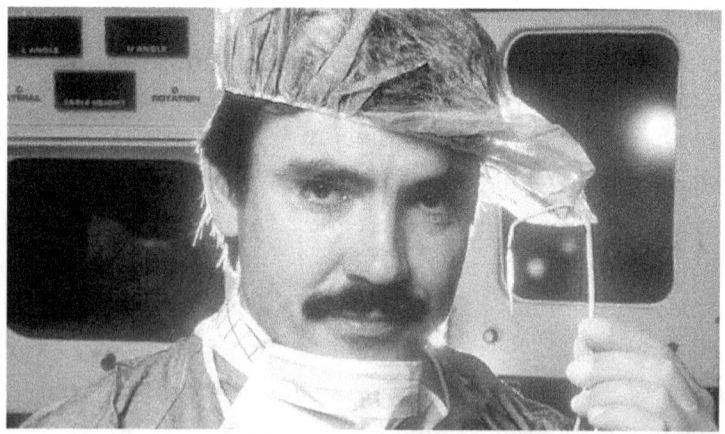

*Fig. 11: Andreas Gruentzig and his balloon catheter*

**Balloon Angioplasty (PTCA):** The oldest and best established procedure is the balloon angioplasty or PTCA (percutaneous transluminal coronary angioplasty). It was first performed by the German cardiologist Andreas Gruentzig in 1977 in Zurich, Switzerland *(see Fig 11)*. Legend has it that the first prototypes of balloon catheters were built on Gruentzig's kitchen table. The procedure reached our shores shortly thereafter, and I am proud to say that I was present at the first procedure done in Philadelphia in the early 1980's, when I was a Cardiology Fellow, although it had been performed in San Francisco and New York years earlier. I met Gruentzig and attended his demonstration course twice before his untimely death in 1985 in a private plane crash (he was an experienced pilot). Andreas Gruenzig was a charismatic personality, that singlehandedly changed the practice of cardiology and vascular medicine forever. He not only invented the technique, but established the criteria for its use, championed it indefatigably throughout the world, demonstrated the scientific validity of its use with a registry where every patient had to be enrolled, and lastly, spread the knowledge with the development of his demonstration courses. Even though these days we tend to call it POBA (poor old balloon angioplasty) in light of the newer and better procedures available, it was a revolution that changed everything. Today, it is still used frequently to prepare the artery for subsequent stenting when the narrowing is so severe that a stent cannot cross without pre-dilating. It is also used to post-dilate after stenting using special non compliant balloons that can withstand inflation with a higher pressure, in order to obtain good apposition of the stent to the vessel wall. It is rarely used as a stand-alone procedure in vessels that are too small to accommodate a stent, or to dilate side branches of bigger arteries that were stented before. Even though the PTCA procedure and the catheters used to perform it have undergone many important improvements, the principle is the same as in the first balloon-tipped catheters built by Gruentzig in his kitchen. The balloon is positioned under X-ray control in the area of stenosis (narrowing of the artery) and inflated with a special device from the outside through a lumen in the catheter, to several times the atmospheric pressure. This pushes the atherosclerotic plaque against the wall of the artery and by squeezing the water out of the plaque, reopens the arterial lumen to reestablish the normal flow of blood to the heart.

Early in the PTCA era it was realized that, even though the procedures were initially successful, tissue tended to grow on the treated area, leading to a phenomenon called restenosis. This occurred in up to 50% of the cases, usually in the first 6 months after treatment, frequently leading to the reappearance of the symptoms that led to the procedure in the first place. Even though the artery could be re-dilated, it was frustrating to patients and doctors alike. Various improvements in technique and pharmacology failed to control the problem. Thus the stent was invented.

**Stent implantation:** This was the next revolution in cardiology. A stent in its simplest form acts as a metallic scaffold that keeps the artery open. Most stents are balloon expandable: mounted on the balloon they are positioned under X-ray control. The balloon is then inflated making the stent expand to the size of the artery and adhere to its wall. Stents not only reduce the incidence of restenosis, as described above, but they keep the artery from collapsing immediately after PTCA. The first stents were approved for use in USA in 1994, initially only for arteries of the legs, and later for coronary arteries. The first stents needed to be crimped on the balloons manually, leading to the not infrequent complication of dislodgement of the stent in the circulation before deployment. The first stents consisted of a metallic mesh shaped in the form of a tube that, when inflating the balloon, would grow to the size of the artery and adhere to it, and upon the deflation of the balloon would stay firmly in place *(see Fig 12)*. These stents, called **bare metal stents**, were made of surgical stainless steel, and were permanent implants. Currently, different space-age alloys are used, such as chromium cobalt, and most stents are coated with different polymers and drugs to further reduce the possibility of restenosis. These are called **drug eluting stents**. Interestingly, it was discovered that the cellular process leading to restenosis is one where the cells of the skin of the artery (endothelium) proliferate out of control, sort of like cancer cells do, eventually leading to the occlusion of the artery. Many of the drugs used to coat the stents are the same as those used for cancer chemotherapy, such as paclitaxel, that slowly incorporate (elute) into the endothelium, keeping it from proliferating. The drugs do not get in the circulation, and therefore do not have the same the toxic effects of chemotherapy. The incidence of restenosis with these stents was reduced to the single digits, to the point where, when repeat cardiac catheterization is required after stent implantation because of recurrent symptoms, we are more frequently finding new areas of stenosis rather than restenosis of the previously stented area.

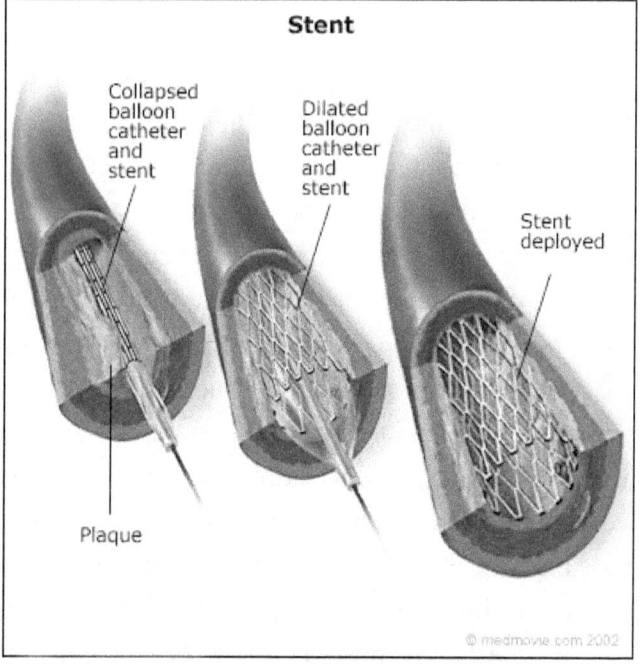

*Fig 12: Stent deployment*

Unfortunately, stents are not able to cure coronary artery disease, and, like many things we do in medicine, they offer only palliation, albeit a very effective one. Stents have evolved since the early days, with novel alloys and designs, thinner struts, and modern drugs, decreasing the incidence of restenosis even further. However, stents are still a permanent implant. The next step in the development of newer devices for the treatment of coronary disease is perhaps the bioabsorbable stent. These are stents that, after deployment, keep the artery from collapsing and release the anti-restenosis drugs. Once done with their mission, they disappear completely. Other devices being tried are drug eluting balloons, obviating the need for stents altogether. Neither of these devices is FDA approved as of this writing, but they are the subject of active research.

**Atherectomy, LASER and other devices:** In the quest for eliminating rather than squashing the atherosclerotic plaques in the coronary arteries, many novel devices have been proposed. Most of these failed to live up to their initial promise, and are no longer in use. We had cooling balloons and hot LASERs, hot balloons and cold LASERs, many of them disastrous and abandoned over time. A form of cold LASER called the Excimer LASER is still in use, mostly for the small arteries of the lower leg. Some so-called atherectomy devices are still in use, in the hopes of cutting or shaving off the plaque. The one that we still use from time to time is the rotational atherectomy (Rotablator), sort of like a dentist's burr that is able to get through very hard, calcified coronary lesions that could not be dilated with a balloon. Other devices, some using ultrasound, have been created to dissolve clots that have produced obstruction of the artery. These are called thrombectomy devices, and there are many different ones in use. Atherectomy and thrombectomy devices are niche products, designed to treat problems that cannot be treated with balloons and stents alone, allowing the successful treatment of blockages in cases where PTCA and stents alone would not work.

There are other devices used during cardiac catheterization and coronary intervention, for diagnostic purposes. These have been reviewed before, namely the intravascular ultrasound (IVUS) and the pressure wire for determination of the fractional flow reserve (FFR). These are used frequently during stent implantation and coronary intervention, both to help determine if stenting is necessary, and to determine the effectiveness of the procedure performed, for example to see if the stent is well apposed to the artery.

Having reviewed the evaluation of chest pain, its various cardiac and non cardiac causes, and the invasive-interventional treatments, it is time now to talk about the medications used to treat CAD.

# Chapter 7

## Drug Treatment of Coronary Artery Disease

*QUICK GUIDE*

*We start this chapter with the drugs used after PTCA and stent deployment, and then proceed to review some of the medications currently used to treat CAD. There is still considerable controversy about the proper place of* **medical therapy versus PTCA and stent deployment**, *and we discuss the pros and cons of each treatment modality in various places in the book. Here, we review the commonly used drugs to treat angina, the chest pain associated with CAD. These include the commonly used* **nitroglycerin**, *the* **beta blockers** *such as metoprolol,* **calcium channel blockers** *such as diltiazem and others: we discuss these drugs, their proper use, the alternatives and some of their side effects. We go over the anti-platelet medications such as* **aspirin and Plavix,** *and also touch on the strategies to reverse or avoid the progression of atherosclerosis. For each person with chest pain, there is a strategy that leads to successful treatment. The information in this chapter will help you discuss these issues with your doctor, who will work with you to find the right combination of medications for your case.*

**For more information or to contact the author, visit** **http://www.tampacardiologist.com.**

This is a very important area. We mentioned before that device therapy of CAD is only palliative, although it is a very effective one. Before we get into the details of pharmacological treatments, let's mention that every patient that receives a stent needs to stay on very powerful clot busting medications, at least for some time. This is because stents, when exposed to the circulation in the artery may promote the activation of platelets, eventually leading to clot formation, a process called **acute or subacute stent thrombosis.** This is a rare but dramatic complication that usually occurs hours or days after stent implantation. Stent thrombosis, if not promptly treated will result in a myocardial infarction. Here again, like in the spontaneously occurring heart attacks, platelets play a central role. Platelets are very interesting cells without a nucleus that circulate in our blood along with the red and white blood cells. They remain inactive while in touch with the smooth, slippery endothelium. But when they encounter something rough, such as the struts of a stent, they may become activated, clumping together and releasing chemicals that eventually will lead to the formation of a thrombus (clot). This is a mechanism of defense of the body, preventing the loss of blood though cuts or injury. When the blood stops circulating, or gets in contact with something that is not the smooth endothelium, the platelets get activated leading to clot formation, and thereby stopping the bleeding. This mechanism of self-preservation becomes a problem when it occurs in the intact but stented artery. Medications used to prevent this from happening by inactivating the platelets are the platelet inhibitors. The most common of these is aspirin, widely used not only to prevent stent thrombosis, but to prevent heart attacks in healthy people (primary prevention), and to treat patients with established CAD. After stent implantation, aspirin needs to be combined with a second, even more powerful platelet inhibitor. The most popular of these medications is **Plavix** or clopidogrel, but there are other two on the market at this writing, **Effient** and **Brilinta**, each with its unique advantages and disadvantages. In spite of their differences, they are similarly effective in preventing stent thrombosis, and one of them will be prescribed for every stent patient. They are necessary for prevention of clot formation on the stent, until this gets "endothelialized," meaning that the endothelium will grow and cover the scent. This takes longer on drug eluting stents (DES) than in bare metal stents (BMS), thus whereas BMS need only one month of double anti-platelet therapy, DES require up to one year. This can be a problem, because these platelet inhibitors increase the risk of bleeding from injuries or during surgery. Many surgeons will not do elective surgery in patients on these drugs, unless they are stopped days or even weeks before surgery. Stopping them, especially early after stent implantation, may lead to life-threatening stent thrombosis, a catch 22 for patients that need surgery.

How about straight drug therapy for CAD, either as an adjuvant to stent implantation, or in lieu of intracoronary intervention? In the last few years there has been a lot of talk about a trial that compared drug therapy for chronic CAD to intervention with balloons and stents. The take home message was that for those patients who respond well to drug treatment, invasive procedures may not offer any advantage. My personal bias, as that of many interventional cardiologists, is that, in patient with demonstrable ischemia (lack of blood supply), especially if they are symptomatic, a well placed stent is not only very effective in relieving those symptoms, but, at least in certain anatomical situations, will decrease the chances of a potentially disabling or even fatal heart attack, with a very low procedural risk. Now, I believe in personalized treatment, and in discussing the options with my patients, but most patients will prefer having a stent to taking lots of medications, and will feel better knowing that their stenosis has been "taken care of." This is not to say that non interventional treatments don't have an important role in our armamentarium and as we saw, stents do not obviate the need for drug treatment.

**Reversal of coronary atherosclerosis:** Many patients ask about reversing CAD, and it is an important question, but a rather elusive goal. We talked already about the importance to achieve a favorable LDL/HDL balance to promote the removal of cholesterol and the possible healing of the atherosclerotic plaque. Many trials of lipid lowering treatments have shown some regression of plaque in the arteries, but we see this very seldom in clinical practice. A very strict and very low-fat, plant based diet, such as that recommended by Dr. Dean Ornish, may attain this goal, but it is very difficult to follow. A reasonable Mediterranean-type diet based on grains and vegetables, healthy oils and fats mostly from fish, and low in refined carbohydrates and red meat, may help prevent progression of plaque. Lowering LDL-cholesterol, the "bad cholesterol" with statin medications, may attain the same goal. Diet and exercise (which may raise the HDL or "good" cholesterol), may help stabilize the coronary plaque and prevent its progression. Anyway, these measures, including food and life-style choices, are always discussed with my patients, before or after stenting or other treatments, and are given great importance, even if they are not the main form of treatment. Given our current understanding of the process, statin medications and diets to reduce LDL-cholesterol are our only hope to reverse CAD.

**Anti-anginal therapy:** Chest pain and equivalent symptoms of angina pectoris have been reviewed before. The treatments directed to decreasing ischemia of the heart muscle and thereby relieving angina, are called anti-anginal therapies. A detailed review of the many anti-anginal agents available is beyond the scope of this book, and if I mention one or another of these preparations, it doesn't mean that I endorse them over others that I didn't mention. As we saw before, angina is produced by a decreased oxygen delivery to the heart, or increased oxygen demand, so we have medications that work on both sides of the equation. The most typical and oldest medication to increase oxygen supply by dilating the arteries is **nitroglycerin**. This compound was first synthesized in the mid-1800's as a dangerous contact explosive, and used extensively in World War I. Alfred Nobel, of the Nobel Prize fame, was its first manufacturer, and also the one to later propose its substitution with the much safer dynamite. Before the end of the 19th century, the medical use of nitroglycerin was described, as a powerful vasodilator.

Nitroglycerine comes in various forms. As a sublingual tablet or in spray form it is absorbed rapidly when placed or sprayed under the tongue, providing immediate relief. There are oral forms of nitrates that are absorbed slowly, providing up to 12 hour protection, and also transdermal preparations to be applied to the skin. In the hospital, we use intravenous nitroglycerin in acute coronary syndromes. We tell our angina patients to always carry sublingual nitro tablets, as they may save the day in case of starting to get angina. Nitroglycerin in this form is absorbed rapidly into the bloodstream from the small vessels under the tongue, and produce dilatation of the coronary arteries within seconds, relieving the symptoms and decreasing the risk of heart attack. The dose can be repeated every 5 minutes, but, if the angina persists after 3 doses, it is time to call 911 and be transported to the emergency room. Sublingual nitroglycerin tablets degrade rapidly in contact with the air once the bottle is opened, and become ineffective. Spray formulations last longer, but are more expensive. Long acting oral preparations, either isosorbide mononitrate tablets or transdermal forms are used to prevent angina attacks before they happen, and get released into the circulation more slowly. All nitroglycerin forms are powerful vasodilators, which is how they relieve ischemia, but they can lower the blood pressure. This can be beneficial though, as it will decrease the need for the heart to pump hard against an elevated blood pressure, and therefore it will not only increase the supply of blood by dilating the coronary arteries, but also decrease the demand of oxygen by decreasing the work of the heart. But, it also may lead to side-effects of lightheadedness, and even fainting.

The other important group of medications is the **beta blockers.** These act by decreasing the work of the heart mostly, but have a number of beneficial effects. They block the beta sympathetic nervous system, a part of the autonomic nervous system of the body, called that way because we have no voluntary control over its functioning. This slows the heart rate and decreases the contractility of the heart muscle, lowering blood pressure. They decrease the incidence and severity of angina episodes in patients with CAD, increasing their exercise capacity and sense of well-being. They are also powerful anti-arrhythmic agents, and exert a so called cardio-protective effect, preventing potentially life threatening heart rhythm disturbances in patients with CAD. They are also known to improve heart function in patients with congestive heart failure. Some popular beta blockers include metoprolol, atenolol, propranolol and others. Most people tolerate beta blockers well, but fatigue, malaise and depression are some of the possible side effects.

A third group are the **calcium channel blockers.**
They are powerful vasodilators and anti-anginal agents,
and some of them are anti-arrhythmic as well. Popular
calcium channel blockers include amlodipine, diltiazem,
verapamil and nifedipine. They are usually well tolerated,
frequently used to lower high blood pressure. A frequent
side effect is ankle swelling or edema, usually mild.

These are the mainstays of anti-anginal therapy,
usually prescribed in combinations of two or more agents
to relieve the symptoms in most sufferers of angina
pectoris. A newer drug called **ranolazine** or Ranexa can
be used in refractory cases, and it works well for some
patients. There are many strategies to avoid angina besides
the drugs reviewed, such as enrolling in an exercise
program to improve the oxygen utilization of the muscles
including perhaps the heart muscle itself. Another strategy
is taking sublingual nitroglycerine before exercise to pre-
dilate the coronary arteries and so prevent angina, or to
take daily aspirin to reduce the chances of clot formation
(although this is not an anti-anginal strategy, it may
prevent an acute cardiac event). For cases where all other
venues have been exhausted and that are not considered
candidates for invasive techniques, there is a mechanical
way to increase the blood flow to the heart, called EECP,
or enhanced external counter pulsation. External air
bladders placed on different parts of the body are inflated
to divert blood to the heart. The results are transient, and
frequent sessions are necessary, making it a time

consuming, less attractive option, with dubious results. Many other methods have been proposed, such as chelation therapy, which has no proven benefit in the treatment of angina, but may be beneficial when heavy metals are involved.

It is important to remember that angina pectoris is a symptom that may be associated with various degrees of coronary involvement, and as many types of pain, it represents a warning. It tells us to stop and rest and to seek medical attention, acting as a safety mechanism. Frequently diabetics have silent ischemia, lacking this safety mechanism. Angina that occurs predictably with a certain level of exercise is what in chapter 3 we called stable angina: this is relatively benign presentation, and is amenable to medical therapy. The treatment is expected to decrease the frequency and severity of the attacks. There is a successful anti-anginal strategy for each person suffering from angina, and the right combination is frequently a matter of trial and error. It is perfectly adequate to try medical treatment in everybody with stable angina, either before we embark on the invasive evaluation or after it. Many cardiologists consider that coronary angiography should be reserved for cases that are refractory to medical therapy, as angiographic evaluation will lead frequently to PTCA and stent implantation. This is a valid approach, but we must be always vigilant. The first sign of unstable angina or acute coronary syndrome, such as when the pain is not promptly relieved with nitroglycerin, or starts occurring more frequently and with less effort, should point us in the direction of the cardiac catheterization laboratory *(see Fig 17)*. This then leads to the interventional treatment options, with balloon angioplasty (PTCA) or stent deployment, or even coronary artery bypass surgery. Whereas there may be some controversy regarding the need and best timing of cardiac catheterization in stable angina, there is very little doubt that, except in some extenuating circumstances, the best option for unstable angina and acute MI is cardiac catheterization. In stable patients that cannot be controlled with medications, cardiac catheterization is also called for in order to define the anatomy. Then, the next decision point is whether to proceed with angioplasty and stent implantation, or in some cases to refer for coronary artery bypass surgery (CABS). We have talked about the former; let us now review the latter.

# Chapter 8

## Coronary Artery Bypass Surgery (CABS)

*QUICK GUIDE*

*This chapter deals with the surgical treatment of CAD. After its creation in 1967, coronary artery bypass surgery (CABS) became the number one surgical procedure performed around the world. Here we describe the* **technique***, and its* **indications***. It is a much more invasive procedure than PTCA, requiring* **open heart** *surgery under general anesthesia, with the heart stopped during the suturing of the grafts and the circulation supported by a heart-lung machine. There are many possible* **complications** *of this complex surgery: the pros and cons of PTCA and stent deployment versus CABS are discussed, including the complications, the time needed for recovery post-op, etc. In spite of all these problems, it is still used in certain cases, and improvements to the technique are being developed. The results are usually longer lasting then those of PTCA and stent, and this main advantage still applies. The discussions in this chapter will provide you with the information you need to discuss these issues with your doctor before you embark on an invasive treatment for your chest pain that may lead to CABS.*

**For more information or to contact the author, visit** *http://www.tampacardiologist.com.*

CABG was the first revolution in the treatment of CAD. The original creation of the technique is attributed to the Argentine surgeon René Favaloro, who performed the first procedure at the Cleveland Clinic in 1967. He was born in a provincial capital, La Plata, and trained as a general surgeon. Early in his career he already showed an interest in the heart. He heard that an American cardiologist, Mason Sones, had developed a technique to selectively visualize the coronary arteries at the Cleveland Clinic in 1963, quite by mistake: he was doing another procedure, and the dye was inadvertently injected into a coronary artery, providing for perfect visualization of the vessel, and without the expected complication of ventricular fibrillation and death. Favaloro had the idea that a vein harvested from the patient's leg called saphenous vein could be used to bypass a coronary blockage, thus providing fresh blood supply to the heart. Precise visualization of the coronary arteries was a must, so he showed up at the Cleveland Clinic, uninvited and with no credentials or qualification, armed only with a good idea and a powerful drive. He was allowed to work in the animal lab, where he was able to demonstrate the feasibility of what came to be known as coronary artery bypass surgery or CABS (sometimes called coronary artery bypass graft or CABG, which is sometimes pronounced "cabbage").

For many years thereafter this procedures was perfected to eventually become the surgical procedure most frequently performed in the world. It is a technically

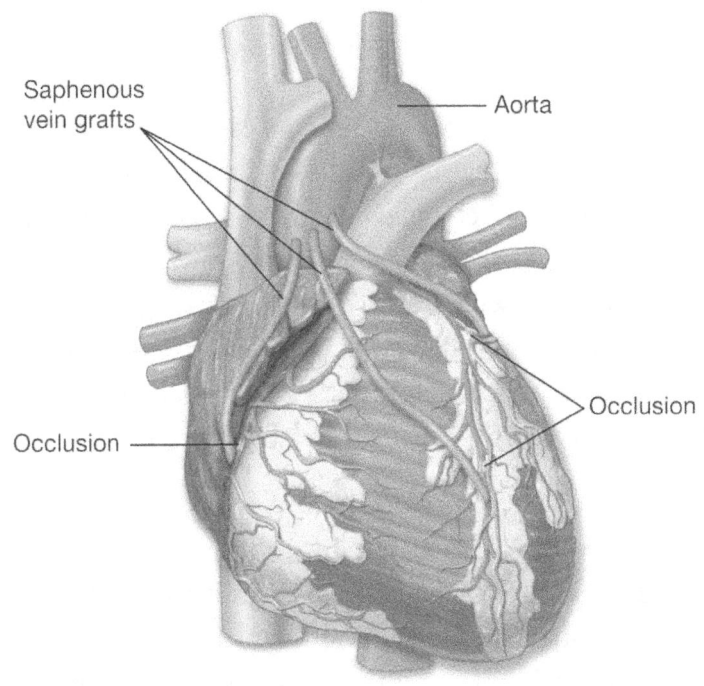

Saphenous
vein grafts

Aorta

Occlusion

Occlusion

*Fig 13: Coronary artery bypass surgery*

demanding operation that proved very successful in relieving the symptoms of angina and keeping patients from having heart attacks, and thereby saving many lives. As it is practiced to this day, veins are harvested from the patient's leg, and inserted between the aorta and the diseased coronary artery, beyond the area of blockage *(see Fig 13)*. These days the artery of the chest wall called the left internal mammary artery (LIMA) is used to bypass the left anterior descending coronary artery (LAD), and frequently other arteries are used to bypass different coronaries, providing for better long-term results than the leg veins. CABS became so popular, and it was so successful, that when angioplasty (PTCA) became available 10 years later as a much less invasive procedure, it took a long time for it to become established. Many of the older cardiologists resisted it, arguing that if we already had a perfectly good therapy (CABS), why should we experiment with something new. It was through the persistence and scientific rigor of Andreas Gruenzig and his followers coupled with the demand of patients for a less invasive procedure, that PTCA and later stent deployment became the most established and frequently used procedure.

**PTCA vs. CABS vs. medical therapy:** So, is CABS an old, obsolete technique destined to disappear? Not so fast, our surgical colleagues tell us. There still are well established indications for the surgical option, and in most trials comparing CABS with PTCA and stenting, CABS offers a longer lasting solution. Even with drug eluting stents, there is still close to 10% chance of restenosis in the first year after stent deployment, requiring repeat procedures. Also, there are subsets of patients where stenting has a higher risk, such as those cases where the stenosis is in the left main coronary artery, where CABS is still the preferred option, at least as far as the accepted guidelines are concerned. The same can be said about triple vessel disease with involvement of the left anterior coronary artery (LAD) in its proximal portions. Also, there is some evidence that diabetic patients may do better with CABG, although many of the studies showing this were done before the advent of drug eluting stents. There are certain areas of the coronary circulation where the incidence of restenosis is higher, such as where one of the main arteries bifurcates, giving off a large branch. In these cases, CABS may be a consideration.

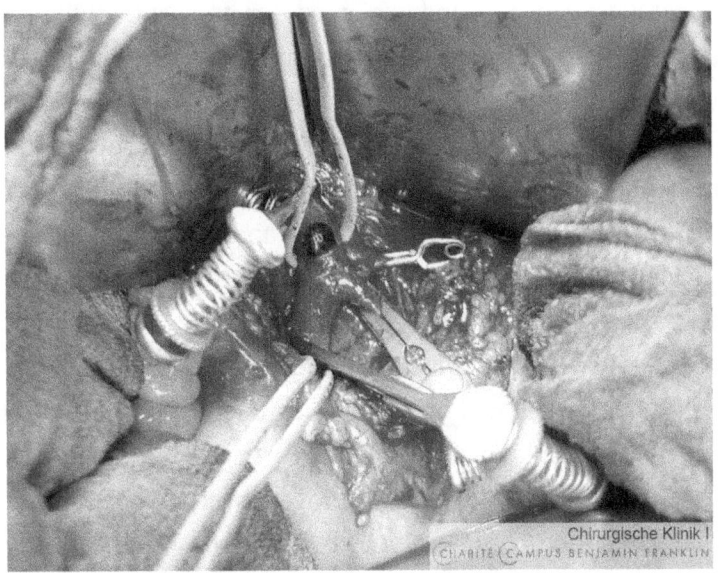

*Fig 14: The exposed heart*

Of course, CABG involves exposing the heart by opening the chest cavity, a much more invasive procedure than PTCA and stent *(see Fig 14)*. The heart needs to be stopped and the circulation sustained with the help of the heart-lung machine during the suturing of the by-pass grafts. CABS involves a certain amount of risk, not only to the heart but to other organs as well. There is considerable discomfort and pain and it usually takes close to a week of in-patient stay (much more if there are complications), and weeks of recovery at home before everything returns to normal and a person can go back to work. The very same patients that may benefit from CABS, such as the diabetics, have more issues with wound healing. Very obese patients have the same and other problems. There are complications inherent to the general anesthesia, and the need for tracheal intubation and the use of mechanical ventilation, particularly in patients with lung problems or sleep apnea. There are sometimes subtle but lasting neurological effects of the heart-lung machine. These and many other problems can be avoided by the use of PTCA and stents, and many times the results are comparable to those with CABG. The only clear-cut advantage of CABG in patients that would be candidates for either procedure is the durability of CABG. The chances of needing a repeat procedure after CABG, particularly in the first few years, are much lower than with PTCA, even considering the very low restenosis rate of modern drug-eluting stents. Since restenosis and progressive CAD are still a possibility after stenting, some patients will require a repeat procedure after some time, usually only years after the first procedure. Stenting can be repeated numerous times if needed. Nobody complains about having to go back to the dentist's office for some additional work, the same may apply to PTCA. Most of us, when given the option, would rather not be intubated with a tube in the trachea and placed on a ventilator, given general anesthesia, have our breastbone split to expose the heart, our heart stopped for several minutes while the bypass grafts are sutured in place, etc. PTCA and stenting do not involve general anesthesia, are non-surgical, there is usually no significant pain involved, the patient goes home the following day and back to work soon thereafter. When given the option, many of us would prefer the less invasive procedure.

Some people think that cardiac catheterization and PTCA are over-utilized in the USA. It is true that lately, in all urban and suburban areas, there are one and sometimes several cardiac units in general hospitals or freestanding centers. These facilities compete for patients, and frequently the pressure is on for the cardiologist to recommend cardiac catheterization sooner or later. Once the anatomy has been defined, it is very easy to succumb to the temptation to intervene with PTCA and stents. In my practice as an invasive-interventional cardiologist, I try to be careful not to give in to the "oculo-dilator reflex," whereby if you see a lesion (blockage), you dilate it. Not all blockages can be dilated, and of those that can, not all need to be so treated. Before we perform a PTCA, most frequently with a permanent implant (stent), we should consider if the patient has received a reasonable medical regimen of drugs, failing to respond. Is her lifestyle severely limited by the symptoms? Is she intolerant or allergic to the proper drugs? Is she at risk of a large heart attack if the artery is not dilated? Can a stent be deployed safely? Are there special anatomical limitations, such as heavy calcium deposits, or very tortuous arteries that would make stent deployment difficult if not impossible? Has ischemia been properly documented, be it with a perfusion scan (nuclear stress test), or with FFR (fractional flow reserve). Is this patient likely to require non-cardiac surgery in the near future, limiting the possibility of taking double anti-platelet therapy? Is there a history of recent bleeding disorder that would preclude the use of double anti-platelet therapy? Is she at high risk for surgery because of systemic diseases? The answers to all these questions and many more help us to settle on a strategy that has the highest chance of success with the lowest possible risk. The guiding principle is always *primum non nocere* (first, do no harm).

# Chapter 9

## Prevention of Cardiovascular Disease

*QUICK GUIDE*

*An ounce of prevention is worth a pound of cure. This most useful chapter for all of us who are at risk of developing CAD deals with prevention of atherosclerosis. In previous chapters we reviewed the process of atherosclerotic plaque formation and the role of cholesterol, as well as the risk factors for the development of CAD. Here we describe **the life-style choices** that lead to the prevention of atherosclerosis, such as **weight loss, diet, exercise and smoking cessation** as well as the more complex problems of the treatment of **lipid disorders** (cholesterol and other lipids), **high blood pressure** (hypertension), and **blood sugar control in diabetes**. These problems, their relation to obesity and their interactions in the **metabolic syndrome**, are analyzed in detail, as well as the treatment options. This chapter is useful even if you have no chest pain (primary prevention), or if you have already established CAD (secondary prevention). Both your primary care physician as well as your cardiologist should discuss these issues with you, and they may suggest further reading material.*

***For more information or to contact the author, visit http://www.tampacardiologist.com.***

So far, we have talked about the risk factors for the development of atherosclerotic disease, the evaluation of chest pain, and the treatment of coronary artery disease. We all know the saying about an ounce of prevention being worth a pound of cure, attributed to Benjamin Franklin. The first order of business is to look objectively at your risk factors. It is rare that somebody without one or more of the known risk factors would develop atherosclerotic disease. Rare, but not impossible. I had one such patient, a 23 year old female nurse complaining of chest pain. She had been seen by one of my partners for her initial evaluation. She did not smoke, had no hypertension or diabetes, had no family history of early atherosclerosis or elevated cholesterol levels. Her risk profile was clearly low, so my partner thought she could wait for further evaluation, as her favorite invasive-interventional cardiologist and herself were both on vacation. I was covering when the young patient presented with intractable chest pain. Cardiac catheterization revealed severe triple vessel coronary artery disease, and a myocardial infarction was threatening to occur at any time. She underwent CABG and recovered uneventfully. A couple of years later she became pregnant, and had a beautiful daughter. A happy ending? Not really, she still had atherosclerotic disease that we did not understand very well, as she lacked the traditional risk factors.

Prevention of atherosclerotic disease is not possible without an understanding of atherogenesis. We already reviewed the classic concepts, namely the development of the fatty infiltration of the arterial wall early in life that, through the years and the exposure to the traditional risk factors results in the formation of the atherosclerotic plaque. Plaques may give no symptoms at all for years until eventually one or several become obstructive and give rise to typical angina pectoris. Sometimes one of these plaques ruptures and exposes its cholesterol laden core to the circulating platelets, resulting in thrombus formation and possibly an acute cardiac event, be it a heart attack or unstable angina. Hence the concept of "vulnerable plaque," a plaque that is likely to rupture. The stable plaque may never rupture, and the plaques that do rupture are not necessarily the ones that grow the most. So, a severe coronary blockage may produce stable angina only, and a less severe plaque may rupture, and give rise to a life-threatening event. How can we recognize such a plaque? What can we do to prevent the rupture of a vulnerable plaque? There is intense research going on in this area, and most of the answers are not in. The focus is on the role of inflammation and thrombogenic factors. For example, an increase in plasma CRP or C-reactive protein, a marker of inflammation, may represent an additional risk factor, or more specifically it may give a warning about the presence of vulnerable plaque. There are invasive methods being developed to identify vulnerable plaques during cardiac catheterization, and perhaps target them for PTCA or stenting to prevent their rupture. While research clarifies some of these issues, we should still focus on the traditional risk factors. As it turns out, smoking cessation, weight loss, control of diabetes, etc, as well as statin medications and aspirin, will lower CRP. Exposure to the traditional risk factors will not only promote the formation of atherosclerotic plaques, but it will also increase their potential to become unstable and rupture. Much can be done to prevent this from happening, be it before plaques even become clinically apparent (primary prevention) or once the plaques are already formed, to retard their growth and so prevent unstable situations (secondary prevention). As we saw before, there is also the possibility of plaque regression, although this is unusual. While there is still much to learn about this subject, we should focus in what we know: the traditional risk factors, and how to manage them.

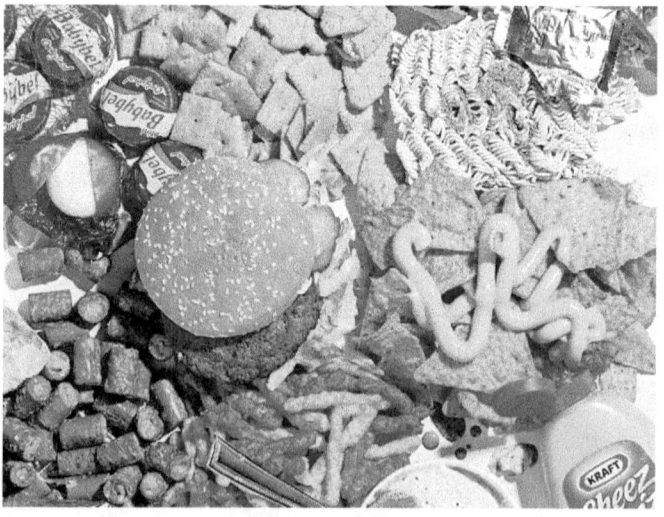

*Fig 15: Junk food*

**Weight loss, diet choices and life-style issues:** A heart healthy diet is low in saturated fats, such as those found in red meat, dairy products (cheese, cream, milk products), and certain vegetable oils such as palm and coconut oils. However, saturated fats are only part of the story. The trans-fatty acids, such as partially hydrogenated vegetable oils found in traditional margarine and vegetable shortening are particularly harmful. Fast food tends to be full of trans-fats or hydrogenated fats, and so are processed foods, commercially baked pastries and cookies, etc. Foods full of these and other harmful chemicals are popularly called junk foods *(see Fig 15)*. A detailed discussion of diet related issues is beyond our scope but the basic principle is to eat as much plant-based foods as possible, replace refined carbohydrates (sugars, baked goods, pasta, potatoes, etc) with whole grain products. If we pay attention to these principles, what we prepare in our kitchen is usually better than what we purchase already made, or what we order at the restaurant. Unsaturated fats, such as the monounsaturated fats found in olive oil, canola oil, avocado, nuts, etc are beneficial. The polyunsaturated fats found in fatty fish are also of great value, probably more so than taking fish oil supplements. If we follow these simple guidelines, we can make sure that our diet is "heart-healthy."

There are many diets and there is a lot of dietary advice out there. We do not advocate any of the "fad diets," as many times their claims of weight loss or lipid lowering are unproven, and some may be even harmful. Weight loss is important if you are obese, but it is certainly not the beginning and the end of prevention of cardiovascular disease by dietary means. We already talked about the "obesity paradox." The content of the diet is as important or more, than the calories consumed *(see Fig 16)*. However, especially in morbid obesity (BMI of 40 or greater), weight loss becomes an important goal in the prevention of heart disease. In these cases, it may be important to seek out professional help, such as that provided by clinical nutritionists or weight loss clinics. Sometimes, obesity by itself is a serious medical condition, and medical help is necessary. For refractory cases, there are surgical options available such as the lap-band procedure, provided by surgeons specializing in bariatric surgery.

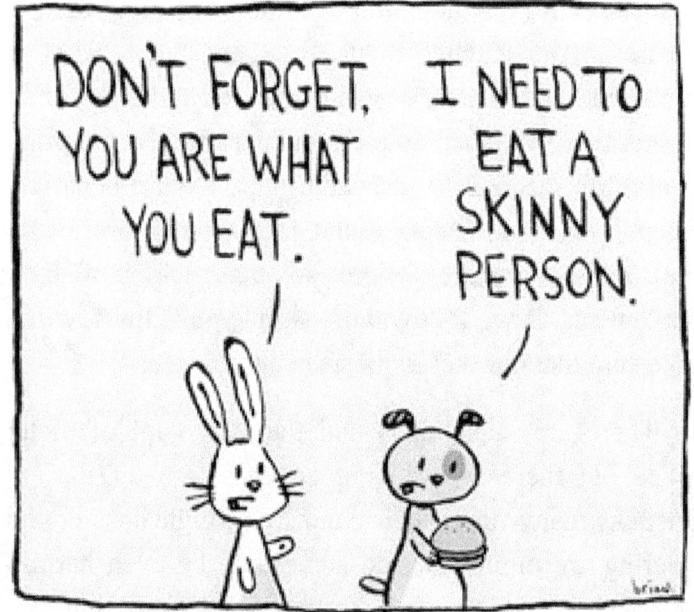

*Fig 16: Good food*

**Exercise** is very important, as a sedentary life-style is a risk factor in itself, as well as a contributor to obesity, hypertension and diabetes. Aerobic exercise, sometimes called "cardio," such as walking, swimming, or any other exercise that involves moving the large muscles is most beneficial. This can be achieved using machines such as the elliptical trainer or the treadmill, or by more natural means such as walking or biking. Anaerobic or resistance exercise, such as weight lifting, may be beneficial for keeping a healthy muscle tone and bone strength, but it adds little cardiovascular benefit. How much exercise do we need, and how strenuous? This is a subject of considerable controversy, but everybody agrees that some exercise is better than none. Ideally, we need close to an hour of sustained exercise at least three or four times a week. How intense? One way of determining the intensity is taking the pulse during exercise. The so-called maximum heart rate is 220 minus your age. We want to keep the heart rate at 70% or so of the maximum heart rate during exercise.

**Control of serum lipids:** We saw how central is cholesterol, particularly LDL-cholesterol in the development of atherosclerotic plaque. Therefore, lowering LDL-cholesterol is one of the most effective means of preventing atherosclerosis. This is particularly true for those of us that have other risk factors, some of which are not amenable to modification. Whether we do it though dietary means, such as those discussed above, or we need to take medications, we should get our LDL as low as possible. These days 100 mg/dl or lower is the "normal" LDL for the general population. If you have other risk factors, such as a family history of early atherosclerosis, the goal is to keep it under 70. Through the years we kept moving the goalpost, requiring lower and lower levels of LDL-cholesterol. Now, these numbers, while desirable, are not always attainable, but the closer we get the lower the risk. Ideally, we should aim to reach the goal by dietary means, but we frequently have to add one or another of the statin medications. Not all medications that lower cholesterol prevent atherosclerosis: Zetia (ezetimibe) lowers cholesterol, particularly when added to a statin, but there is no proof that it will prevent cardiac events. The statins (rosuvastatin, atorvastatin, lovastatin and others) have been proven to do both, lower LDL-cholesterol and lower the risk of a cardiac event. Common side effects include muscle aches, and uncommon but serious toxicity may include elevation of liver enzymes and muscle damage, etc.

Other lipid fractions in the blood include HDL, the "good cholesterol," and triglycerides. Actually, HDL is only good because, as we saw before, it transports cholesterol to the liver to be metabolized, making it unavailable to the arterial wall, and therefore reducing the risk of atherosclerosis. Low HDL seems to be an independent risk factor. We want to keep HDL-cholesterol above 40 mg/dl. If you have low HDL-cholesterol there is really not a consistently effective treatment. A sedentary lifestyle and smoking tend to lower HDL, and should be addressed. Niacin (nicotinic acid) and fibrates like gemfibrozil and fenofibrate may raise HDL modestly. Triglycerides are another lipid fraction, and they should be kept under 150 mg/dl. They may be lowered with the same medications that are used to raise HDL. In addition, omega-3 fatty acids contained in fish oil may help, although eating oily fish such as salmon is even better. Triglycerides follow serum glucose, and in diabetics strict control of blood sugar helps to lower triglycerides.

We have not discussed other, more subtle issues related to hyperlipidemia, such as the importance of LDL-cholesterol particle size. Some specialized laboratories are able to sub fractionate LDL, and the most atherogenic and thrombogenic are the small, dense particles. Lowering triglycerides and increasing HDL-cholesterol may help increasing the particle size of LDL, thus making it less harmful. Other fractions such as Lp(a) or lipoprotein(a) are also atherogenic. Routine lab tests do not include sub-fractionation of LDL or the measurement of Lp(a), and these sophisticated tests are only useful in special situation, such as when the risk profile is otherwise unclear. In most people, a routine lipid profile will suffice, including total cholesterol, LDL (direct measurement) and HDL cholesterol and triglycerides. Calculated LDL is inaccurate and should not be used, especially in cases where the triglycerides are high such as in diabetics.

**Diabetic control:** Diabetes is probably the strongest risk factor for the development of atherosclerotic vascular disease. The probability of having an acute cardiovascular event is as high in diabetics without a previous history of atherosclerotic disease, as it is in non-diabetics with already established atherosclerotic disease. So, diabetes is said to be an "atherosclerotic equivalent" risk factor.

Normally glucose, a simple sugar is transported in the blood stream to the tissues, where it is metabolized with the help of insulin. Glucose, either from the diet or from storage sites is used as a source of energy by most organisms. Insulin is a hormone produced by the pancreas, and it is necessary for the metabolism of glucose. Diabetes mellitus is a disorder of glucose metabolism, characterized by the presence of elevated concentration of serum glucose or "blood sugar." The most frequent form is type II diabetes, where there is normal secretion of insulin by the pancreas, but the tissues that are supposed to utilize and metabolize the glucose become resistant to insulin. The tissues cannot metabolize glucose and therefore it accumulates in the blood. This insulin resistance goes hand in hand with obesity, although not all diabetics are obese. Type I diabetes, a less common form, is a totally different disease: here the high blood sugar is caused by a deficiency in the production of insulin itself, and obesity does not play a role. Type I diabetes used to be called juvenile diabetes, as it tends to have its onset early in life.

Measurement of fasting blood sugar, and of glycosylated hemoglobin, (the so-called hemoglobin A1c or HbA1c), should be included in every assessment of atherosclerotic risk, and should be repeated frequently in diabetics to assess the adequacy of the treatment. An elevated HbA1c means that the blood sugar has been frequently above normal in the preceding months. Blood sugar in non-diabetics is less than 100 mg/dl and normal HbA1c is less than 5.7; these are also the goals of the treatment in diabetics. Strict control of blood sugar along with effective control of other associated risk factors, is necessary to improve the chances of delaying the development of symptoms of atherosclerotic disease (such as MI or stroke) in this common disease.

Diabetes is treated with diet and medications. The diabetic diet is low in carbohydrates, especially refined carbohydrates and sugar itself. Whereas type I diabetics always require injected insulin (the only route available for this protein, that would be degraded if taken orally), type II diabetics may do with oral medications such as the popular **metformin**, usually in combination with sulfonylureas like **glyburide** or others. Once advanced, type II diabetes also is treated with various forms of **insulin**, usually injected under the skin several times a day.

**Metabolic syndrome**. Most of the modifiable risk factors are associated with one another, and there are common forms of management. Obesity is a harbinger of type II diabetes, as it promotes insulin resistance. Exercise and weight loss are very helpful in controlling blood sugar in diabetes and blood pressure in hypertension. Triglycerides "follow" blood sugar, and in fact, the diet to lower triglycerides is the same low sugar and low refined carbohydrate diet used in diabetes. A so called **metabolic**

**syndrome** has been described: it consists of elevated blood sugar, low HDL-cholesterol, high triglycerides, hypertension, and obesity, particularly the so-called central obesity characterized by increased waist size. There are many different definitions and cut-off points, but these are the basic criteria for the diagnosis of the syndrome. Obesity and insulin resistance are the central features. The metabolic syndrome is a recognized risk factor for atherosclerotic disease and coronary events. Control of body weight and blood sugar, treatment of hypertension and lipid disorder may reverse the cardiovascular risk associated with the metabolic syndrome.

**Smoking cessation:** By now, everybody knows about the damaging effects of smoking, and we will not discuss them here in detail. Smoking promotes the formation of atherosclerotic plaques in the arteries, leading to heart attacks, strokes and peripheral vascular disease, particularly of the arteries of the legs. The risk of such diseases is 2 to 4 times higher in smokers than nonsmokers. More than 400,000 deaths per year are directly attributable to smoking, and is the number one killer in the whole world from cardiovascular disease, emphysema and cancer, mostly of the lung. Smoking not only promotes plaque formation, but it elevates blood pressure, increases the oxygen consumption of the heart while it decreases the supply, it constricts the blood vessels, it promotes clotting, etc. Both nicotine as well as other substances released by the burning of tobacco and fillers, such as carbon monoxide, are deleterious, whether you smoke or are exposed to second hand smoke. Smoking has immediate effects: smoking just one cigarette immediately elevates heart rate and blood pressure, constricts blood vessels, decreases the oxygen in the blood, promotes clotting, etc, increasing the risk of ischemia. The nicotine contained in cigarette replacement products, such as nicotine gums and transdermal patches, and more recently electronic cigarettes, has much of the same effects, but may help in quitting while avoiding the exposure to smoke itself.

**Blood pressure control:** Last but not least, high blood pressure is another major modifiable risk factor. Of course, like with smoking, the problem is not only the increased formation of plaque, but dangerously elevated blood pressure may lead to the rupture of an aneurysm in the aorta, or to a stroke, both potentially life threatening conditions. Blood pressure above the normal of 120/80 needs to be treated. Initially, many will try with salt restriction, weight loss and exercise, which are all of paramount importance to control blood pressure. Frequently drug therapy needs to be added when blood pressure cannot be controlled by diet and exercise. There are numerous drugs for blood pressure control that we will not discuss here. The treatment is hit or miss, whatever works to lower blood pressure is good. The election of the drug sometimes rests on other conditions that the person may have, such as the cardio-protective effect of beta blockers **(atenolol, metoprolol, carvedilol** and many others) in coronary artery disease. Others, such as the angiotensine converting enzyme (ACE) inhibitors such as **lisinopril and enalapril** for example, may have renal protective effects.

Most of the time hypertension is "primary," meaning that a specific cause cannot be found. When there is a cause, this needs to be treated, such as some cases of hormonal imbalance. Sometimes "secondary" hypertension is related to atherosclerotic blockage of the arteries feeding the kidneys, the renal arteries. In these cases, stenting those arteries may help to bring blood pressure back to normal. Hypertension is more frequent in African-Americans and Asians, and the treatment frequently involves a combination of several drugs. How low do we want the blood pressure? As close to normal as possible. The lower the blood pressure, the greater the life expectancy.

So these are the risk factors that we need to control in order to prevent the development and progression of heart disease and atherosclerosis. There are others, such as gender and age that we have no control over. As we saw, family history is important, but we don't get to pick our ancestors and siblings. So, the measures reviewed above are those that we can put in practice to prevent the development or the progression of atherosclerotic disease of the coronary arteries leading to heart attacks, or of the carotid arteries leading to strokes. We have not talked much about **peripheral arterial disease (PAD)** and its symptoms, as we have focused on heart disease, but atherosclerosis affects all the arteries of the body. When affecting the arteries of the legs, it may lead to a symptom called intermittent claudication, a crampy pain generally of the calf muscles, occurring during exercise such as walking, and relieved with rest. It is frequently a harbinger of coronary artery disease, and it is frequently treated with angioplasty and stents, just like coronary artery disease. Atherosclerosis of the renal arteries may lead to renal failure and uncontrolled hypertension, and those of the intestines to abdominal pain or even acute, life threatening abdominal events such as bowel ischemia. Same can be said about atherosclerotic disease of the carotid arteries and its relation with strokes. These problems are beyond the scope of this book, and I mention them only because they are frequently associated with atherosclerotic disease of the coronary arteries and chest pain. They respond to the same risk factors, and the same preventative measures as for coronary artery disease, and frequently the invasive treatment is similar, with the use of balloons and stents. Many interventional cardiologists like myself are trained to perform procedures in the peripheral arteries as well.

# Chapter 10

## Do I Have CAD? A Useful Algorithm

*QUICK GUIDE*

*Heart attack or indigestion? This was our original question, that now we are much better equipped to answer, after having read our previous chapters. In this chapter we develop a **point system** that first considers the **risk factors** that we may have, such as age and gender, lipid disorders, diabetes, family history, obesity and smoking. Then, it considers the **symptoms**, their relation with effort, etc, adding more points, or subtracting if an alternative explanation for the symptoms exist. Then we simply add the points, and voila, we have an answer to the original question. Well, it would be nice if it were as simple as that, but unfortunately the answer is not white or black, there are many gray areas. We analyze some particular cases, and try to come up with some good answers, but like always, these consideration are just a springboard to dive into these subject with your doctor, who will consider your whole situation and recommend further testing if necessary, as well as the proper treatment.*

***For more information or to contact the author, visit** http://www.tampacardiologist.com.*

We come back to our initial question, now armed with the knowledge acquired during the reading of the preceding chapters. I assume you read the whole thing and didn't just take a short-cut here, did you? Hopefully, having read about the diagnosis and treatment of atherosclerotic coronary artery disease, you are now much better qualified to answer the question posed in the title, or are you? It is a bit confusing, and the answers are frequently not cut and dry. Let us see if we can make some sense of all this knowledge. I am going to propose an algorithm, with 10 simple questions to ask yourself, and a score assigned to each yes or no answer, then we'll add the points to determine your likelihood of having coronary artery disease. Some of the cutoff points are arbitrary, and some of the answers are purely subjective, but there it goes. The premise, of course, is that you are having chest pain, and you are not sure if it is related to coronary artery disease, and if you are at risk of having a heart attack.

1. Assign two point to each of the major risk factors: smoking, elevated LDL-cholesterol, diabetes, family history of early atherosclerosis, hypertension and obesity. You only need to assign one point to each risk factor if it is well controlled, or in the case of smoking, if you quit some time ago.

2. Add a point if you are male, or post menopausal female.

3. Add another point if you are 65 years old or older.

4. Add another point if you had an elevated calcium

score on a CT scan of your heart.

5. Add one point if you have a low HDL-cholesterol, or high triglycerides, or a high C-reactive protein on your blood test, or if you are "pre-diabetic," (impaired glucose tolerance), or are overweight but not obese (BMI over 27 but less than 30) or if you are sedentary. These risk factors may be additive (if you have more than one, add a point for each).

6. Add 2 points if you have already established atherosclerotic disease: this may be a history of stroke, or peripheral arterial disease, or of course, if you have established coronary artery disease.

7. Add 5 points if your chest pain is related to exercise or effort, and relieved by rest.

8. Add 5 extra point if you have typical symptoms: an aching type of pain, not sharp, located in the mid chest area and radiating to the left shoulder neck or jaw, not exacerbated by a certain movement or a certain body position, not related to the respiratory cycle or taking a deep breath, not reproducible by pressing on the area.

9. Subtract 2 points if you have an alternative explanation for your chest pain, such as gastro-esophageal reflux, a pulled muscle or joint pain, costochondritis, trauma, etc. Of course, having an alternative explanation is no warranty against developing ischemic heart disease, as you may have more than one kind of chest pain.

10. Add one point if you were examined by a doctor or nurse, and "nothing was found" or you were given a "clean bill of health." Just joking, but most of the time this

is the case in coronary artery disease, there are no obvious findings on a routine examination.

There you have it. Simple, is it not? Let's say we have a non-smoking, non diabetic 65 year old male who walks an hour at least 3 times a week (2 points for age and gender), with a treated lipid disorder and an LDL of 110, HDL of 45 and triglycerides of 145 (2 points for high LDL), with BMI of 32 (2 points for obesity), with controlled hypertension (one point), who developed chest pain that is on the right upper chest, constant, made worse by rotating the shoulder. There is no typical chest pain during exercise. That adds up to 7 points so far. Ah, and that is me, after painting the ceiling in my house, so I can subtract 2 points for having an alternative explanation for my chest pain. Am I on my way of having a heart attack, with 5 points? I hope not, and having atypical symptoms and an alternative explanation for those symptoms, should reassure me that I am not having a heart attack, but if I could control my risk factors better, like for example losing some weight, my score could improve a lot. So can we say that a score of 5 or less represents low risk, a score of 6 to 10 is intermediate risk, and a score of 10 or higher is high risk? Well, that sounds good but is only an educated guess, the result of an oversimplified algorithm.

How many points do you need to make the diagnosis of coronary artery disease? I wish it were as simple as counting points. If that would be the beginning and the end of diagnosing coronary artery disease, we would need no cardiologists or any of the testing methods described in earlier chapters. Unfortunately, coronary artery disease is a treacherous disease, it may be dormant for years and then progress rapidly to a heart attack or it may be totally silent and present after an undiagnosed heart attack, once heart failure develops. I have seen many examples of all these presentations, as well as patients with a very low risk profile who present with severe disease, as the young nurse I talked about before, and others with all the risks who never develop any disease at all. In clinical practice it is not unusual to see patients to present with totally atypical symptoms that then go away once their coronary artery disease is corrected. I cannot tell you if there is a safe cut-off point, below which you can be reasonably assured that your pain is not related to heart disease. It is a continuum, and the more points you accumulate, the higher the likelihood that you are having a cardiac problem, but there is not a well defined borderline between non-cardiac chest pain and coronary artery disease. And of course, if you are having unrelenting chest pain, especially if you have some telltale associated symptoms such as shortness of breath, nausea, profuse sweating or palpitations, you may be having a heart attack or unstable angina, and all bets are off. You need to call 911 and get emergency help. Short of that emergency, there is a spectrum of cardiac or non-cardiac problems that can be better elucidated by a visit to the cardiologist and proper testing. As we saw, some non-cardiac conditions may also be life-threatening, and need to be diagnosed before they can cause problems.

# Chapter 11

## How to Pick a Cardiologist

---

*QUICK GUIDE*

*Like in the talk shows we finish with a plug. In this case, it is for selecting the best cardiologist for you when you are experiencing chest pain. First, consider the recommendations of your primary care physician; he or she knows you best. When it comes to selecting the right cardiologist, consider their **training and credentials**, their **reputation in the community**, their **hospital affiliations**, etc. Don't be afraid to ask questions. Not only should your cardiologist have credentials but also "people skills" to dedicate time to listen to your complaints and try to understand your unique background. Lastly, you should consider all the diagnostic and treatment procedures that may apply to your case: if your main problem is your cholesterol and risk factor management you may pick a **lipid specialist**, or you may want a **cardiac electrophysiologist** for your heart rhythm problem. But if you have chest pain, and you want somebody with the greatest knowledge about the anatomy and pathology of the cardiovascular system who can help you get to the bottom of the problem, you should pick somebody with the broadest and deepest training background: **an invasive-interventional cardiologist.***

***For more information or to contact the author, visit** http://www.tampacardiologist.com.*

---

To finish, let me make a comment about the state of our profession that may help you pick the right professional to diagnose and treat your possible heart condition. As everybody knows, to become a doctor takes many years of difficult and absorbing training, so many professionals graduate with the technical skills but without the so called "people skills" of empathy and communication to be a good doctor. Some of these skills cannot be taught in school, you either have them, or you don't. Listen to the recommendations of your friends and neighbors, they know which doctor listened to them and took the time to understand not only their symptoms but their circumstances. How about those technical skills? Should you find out if they graduated of a first tier medical school, or how many years of training do they have? Not necessarily, although it may help. One of the best cardiologists I know, a friend of mine, graduated from medical school in Grenada, and did his post graduate training in Coney Island, NY, not a very distinguished background, I would say. Yet he is a great professional, with all the requisite skills that you or anybody would need to diagnose and treat heart disease. Many doctors trained in Ivy League schools are not nearly as good as my friend, and I would not hesitate to pick him as my cardiologist. I would recommend that you make sure that the cardiologist you are going to see is a fellow of the American College of Cardiology, denoted by the initials FACC after their name. That means that they are fully trained and passed all the required Board exams, which is a minimum requirement. Beyond that, I would check if they hold admitting privileges at your local hospital, preferably one with full cardiac services including invasive diagnostic and interventional capabilities, such as a cardiac catheterization laboratory with interventional credentialing *(see Fig 17)*. There are many web sites that keep track of doctor's reputations, but in my experience they are not very reliable, as they are based on patient reports, many times just a few. A disgruntled patient is much more likely to report a doctor than a satisfied one, and it is relatively easy to stuff a site with good or bad reports from friends or enemies respectively. Of course, if they have been disciplined by the Board of Professional Regulation, or had their license suspended, that would be a big warning sign. If they have been found guilty of malpractice, this could be a problem as well.

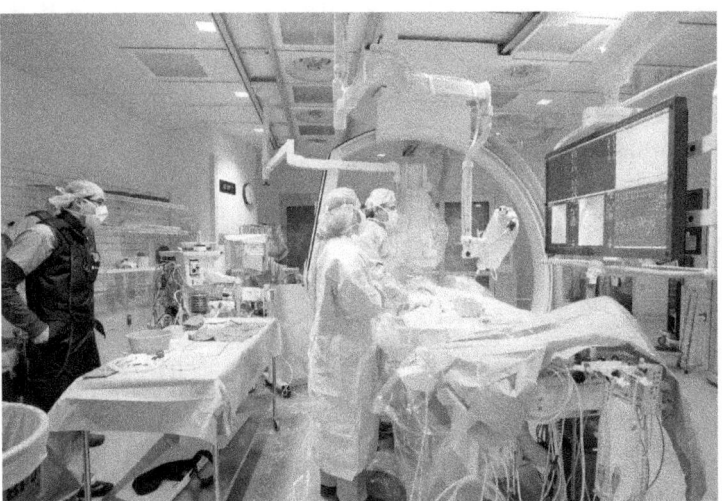

*Fig 17: Cardiac catheterization lab*

Many cardiologists specialize in areas of cardiology that may be of interest to you. This may include invasive and interventional cardiology, peripheral vascular disease, cardiac electrophysiology, heart failure and transplantation, lipid disorders, etc. These sub-specialties require additional training, sometimes one or more years. For example, an invasive and interventional cardiologist that also specializes in the treatment of peripheral vascular disease will have four years of college, another four years of medical school, three years of internal medicine residency, three years of cardiology fellowship, and at least one and frequently two more years of sub-specialty training. All this training, assuming they pass all the Board exams, allows them to diagnose and treat a wide variety of cardiac and vascular conditions, including all areas of clinical and diagnostic cardiology, as well as coronary and peripheral angiography and angioplasty, the use of various intravascular diagnostic and therapeutic methods that we describe in this book, and the implantation of stents and other devices in the circulation. Should you pick one of these highly trained cardiologists for your evaluation, if you have chest pain or think you may have some cardio-vascular problems? Well, yes, depending on the issues you want addressed. Many problems can be addressed by your family doctor or internist. Your problem may be control of your cholesterol, and a lipid specialist may be best, or you may have a heart rhythm disorder best evaluated and treated by a cardiac electrophysiologist. But if you have chest pain, and you want somebody with the vastest knowledge about the anatomy and pathology of the cardiovascular system who can help you get to the bottom of the problem, you might as well pick somebody with the broadest and deepest training background: an invasive-interventional cardiologist. Your chest pain may just be indigestion, but I bet you would feel better if the diagnosis is made after exhausting all the other possibilities, by a highly trained professional that knows your heart inside out.

The purpose of this book is never to replace a proper consultation with your physician: in my experience self-diagnosis is always problematic even if you are a cardiologist yourself. But that doesn't mean that a person with chest pain shouldn't have access to as much knowledge as possible. If the information in this book could help you in any way to make the right decisions about your cardiovascular health, I have accomplished my goal.

# ABOUT THE AUTHOR

Dr. Roberto P. Medina MD is a practicing clinical invasive-interventional cardiologist with more than 30 years of experience seeing patients with chest pain every day in his offices, and performing invasive and interventional procedures. He is also a family man with two adult children and 35 years of marriage. He is an avid traveler and an accomplished photographer and has published several books of photography.

**Visit http://www.tampacardiologist.com for more information!**

www.ingramcontent.com/pod-product-compliance
Lightning Source LLC
Chambersburg PA
CBHW051330170526
45166CB00002B/749